BLUEPRINTS
Ophthalmology

Blueprints **for your pocket!**

In an effort to answer a need for high yield review books for the elective rotations, Blackwell Publishing now brings you Blueprints in pocket size.

These new Blueprints provide the essential content needed during the shorter rotations. They will also provide the basic content needed for USMLE Steps 2 and 3, or if you were unable to fit in the rotation, these new pocket-sized Blueprints are just what you need.

Each book will focus on the high yield essential content for the most commonly encountered problems of the specialty. Each book features these special appendices:

- Career and residency opportunities
- Commonly prescribed medications
- Self-test Q&A section

Ask for these at your medical bookstore or check them out online at www.blackwellmedstudent.com

Blueprints Dermatology
Blueprints Urology
Blueprints Pediatric Infectious Diseases
Blueprints Ophthalmology
Blueprints Plastic Surgery
Blueprints Orthopedics
Blueprints Hematology and Oncology
Blueprints Anesthesiology
Blueprints Infectious Diseases
Blueprints Gastroenterology

BLUEPRINTS
Ophthalmology

Thomas E. Bournias, MD
Director
Northwestern Ophthalmic Institute
Assistant Clinical Professor
Department of Ophthalmology
Northwestern University Feinberg School of Medicine
Chicago, Illinois

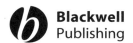

Blackwell
Publishing

© 2005 by Blackwell Publishing

Blackwell Publishing, Inc., 350 Main Street, Malden, Massachusetts 02148-5018, USA
Blackwell Publishing Ltd, 9600 Garsington Road, Oxford OX4 2DQ, UK
Blackwell Publishing Asia Pty Ltd, 550 Swanston Street, Carlton, Victoria 3053, Australia

04 05 06 07 5 4 3 2 1

ISBN: 1-4051-0440-6

Library of Congress Cataloging-in-Publication Data

Bournias, Thomas E.
    Blueprints ophthalmology/Thomas E. Bournias.
        p. ; cm.
    Includes bibliographical references and index.
    ISBN 1-4051-0440-6 (alk. paper : pbk.)
    1. Ophthalmology—outlines, syllabi, etc. 2. Eye—Diseases—outlines, syllabi, etc.
    I. Title. II. Title: Ophthalmology.
    [DNLM: 1. Eye Diseases—Handbooks. 2. Diagnostic Techniques, Ophthalmological—Handbooks. 3. Eye Injuries—Handbooks.
    4. Ophthalmologic Surgical Procedures—Handbooks. WW 39 B775b 2005]
    RE50.B685 2005
    617.7—dc22

                                                            2004014746

A catalogue record for this title is available from the British Library

Acquisitions: Beverly Copland
Development: Selene Steneck
Production: Debra Murphy
Cover design: Hannus Design Associates
Interior design: Mary McKeon
Illustrations: Electronic Illustrators Group
Typesetter: International Typesetting and Composition, Ft. Lauderdale, FL
Printed and bound by Capital City Press in Berlin, VT

For further information on Blackwell Publishing, visit our website:
www.blackwellmedstudent.com

Notice: The indications and dosages of all drugs in this book have been recommended in the medical literature and conform to the practices of the general community. The medications described do not necessarily have specific approval by the Food and Drug Administration for use in the diseases and dosages for which they are recommended. The package insert for each drug should be consulted for use and dosage as approved by the FDA. Because standards for usage change, it is advisable to keep abreast of revised recommendations, particularly those concerning new drugs.

For Olympia

My wonderful wife and mother of our beautiful children, Evalina and Efthimios. You give me great happiness and make all my professional work possible.

Contents

Chapter 12: Common Ocular Surgery 166
Thomas E. Bournias, MD and Jerry Lai, MD

Contributors

Charlie Abraham, MD
Postdoctoral Fellow, Department of Ophthalmology
Northwestern University Feinberg School of Medicine
Chicago, Illinois

Anthony Cirino, MD
Fellow, Department of Ophthalmology
Northwestern University Feinberg School of Medicine
Chicago, Illinois

Jerry Lai, MD
Resident, Department of Ophthalmology
Northwestern University Feinberg School of Medicine
Chicago, Illinois

Preeya Kshettry, BS
Class of 2006
Northwestern University Feinberg School of Medicine
Chicago, Illinois

P. Oat Sinchai, MD
Resident, Department of Ophthalmology
Georgetown University Medical Center
Washington, DC

Angie E. Wen, MD
Housestaff Physician, Department of Ophthalmology
Summa Health System
Akron City Hospital
Akron, Ohio

Photography Consultant

Jonathan Shankle, CRA
Department of Ophthalmology
Northwestern University Feinberg School of Medicine
Chicago, Illinois

Reviewers

Shanti Bansal
Class of 2004
Rush Medical College
Chicago, Illinois

Rachel Shemtov
Class of 2004
Yale Medical School
New Haven, Connecticut

Sean Armin, MD
Resident in Neurological Surgery
Loma Linda University Medical Center
Loma Linda, California

John Nguyen, MD
PGY-I, Internal Medicine Prelim/Ophthalmology
University of Texas Medical Branch
Galveston, Texas

Kevin N. Sheth, MD
Resident, Partners Neurology
Brigham and Women's Hospital/Massachusetts General Hospital
Harvard Medical School
Boston, Massachusetts

Preface

Blueprints have become the standard for medical students to use during their clerkship rotations and sub-internships and as a review book for taking the USMLE Steps 2 and 3.

Blueprints initially were only available for the five main specialties: medicine, pediatrics, obstetrics and gynecology, surgery, and psychiatry. Students found these books so valuable that they asked for Blueprints in other topics and so family medicine, emergency medicine, neurology, cardiology, and radiology were added.

In an effort to answer a need for high yield review books for the elective rotations, Blackwell Publishing now brings you Blueprints in pocket size. These books are developed to provide students in the shorter, elective rotations, often taken in 4th year, with the same high yield, essential contents of the larger Blueprint books. These new pocket-sized Blueprints will be invaluable for those students who need to know the essentials of a clinical area but were unable to take the rotation. Students in physician assistant, nurse practitioner, and osteopath programs will find these books meet their needs for the clinical specialties.

Feedback from student reviewers gave high praise for this addition to the Blueprints brand. Each of these new books was developed to be read in a short time period and to address the basics needed during a particular clinical rotation. Please see the Series Page for a list of the books that will soon be in your bookstore.

Acknowledgments

I would like to express my many thanks to all the people who made this book possible. My sincerest thanks to my family for their love, understanding and continuous support throughout this endeavor. I would also like to thank Daniel T. Weidenthal, MD, my mentor, for providing inspiration and demonstrating how we as physicians should strive to give the highest level of compassion and care to our patients. Many thanks to Martin S. Lipsky, MD for his invaluable advice and to Cynthia Walter for her exemplary contributions in organizing and preparing this manuscript. Many thanks to Lee Jampol, MD and the Department of Ophthalmology at Northwestern University's Feinberg School of Medicine for providing a stimulating academic environment. And finally, thanks to Beverly Copland, Selene Steneck and all of the editorial staff at Blackwell Publishing for making this work possible.

—Thomas E. Bournias, MD

Abbreviations

AC	anterior chamber
ACE	angiotensin-converting enzyme
ACGME	Accreditation Council for Graduate Medical Education
ACG	angle-closure glaucoma
AK	astigmatic keratotomy
ALT	argon laser trabeculoplasty
AMD	age-related macular degeneration
ANA	antinuclear antibody
ANCA	antineutrophilic cytoplastic antibody
APD	afferent pupillary defect
AVN	arteriovenous nicking
BDR	background diabetic retinopathy
BRAO	branch retinal artery occlusion
BRVO	branch retinal vein occlusion
CBC	complete blood count
CCT	central corneal thickness
C/F	cell and flare
CME	cystoid macular edema
CMV	cytomegalovirus
CN	cranial nerve
CNS	central nervous system
CNV	choroidal neovascularization
CNVM	choroid neovascular membrane
CRAO	central retinal artery occlusion
CRVO	central retinal vein occlusion
CSME	clinically significant macular edema (in diabetes)
CT	computed tomography
CVF	confrontational visual field
CWS	cotton-wool spot
DFE	dilated fundus examination
DR	diabetic retinopathy
ECCE	extracapsular cataract extraction
EOM	extraocular muscle
ERD	exudative retinal detachment
ERG	electroretinogram
ERM	epiretinal membrane
ESR	erythrocyte sedimentation rate
EUA	examination under anasthesia
FB	foreign body

FTA-ABS	fluorescent treponemal antibody, absorbed
GCA	giant cell arteritis
GPC	giant papillary conjunctivitis
HLA	human leukocyte antigen
HRT	Heidelberg retinal tomography
HSV	herpes simplex virus
HVF	Humphrey visual field
HZO	herpes zoster ophthalmicus
HZV	herpes zoster virus
ICCE	intracapsular cataract extraction
IK	interstitial keratitis
INO	internuclear ophthalmoplegia
IOL	intraocular lens
IOP	intraocular pressure
KS	Krukenberg spindle
LASIK	laser-assisted in situ keratomileusis
LGN	lateral geniculate nucleus
LPI	laser peripheral iridotomy
MRI	magnetic resonance imaging
MS	multiple sclerosis
NAG	narrow-angle glaucoma
NFL	nerve fiber layer
NPDR	nonproliferative diabetic retinopathy
NVD	neovascularization of the disc
NVE	neovascularization elsewhere (of the retina)
NVG	neovascular glaucoma
NVI	neovascularization of the iris
OCT	ocular coherence tomography
PAS	peripheral anterior synechia
PDR	proliferative diabetic retinopathy
PDS	pigment dispersion syndrome
PDT	photodynamic therapy
PEX	pseudoexfoliation
PHPV	persistent hyperplastic primary vitreous
PI	peripheral iridectomy
POAG	primary open-angle glaucoma
PPA	peripapillary atrophy
PPD	purified protein derivative
PPV	pars plana vitrectomy
PRK	photorefractive keratectomy
PRP	panretinal photocoagulation
PVR	proliferative vitreoretinopathy
PXE	pseudoexfoliation
RK	radial keratotomy
RAPD	relative afferent pupillary defect
RBC	red blood cell
RD	retinal detachment
ROP	retinopathy of prematurity

RPE	retinal pigment epithelium
RPR	rapid plasma reagin (test)
RRD	rhegmatogenous retinal detachment
SDP	stereo disc photos
SLT	selective laser trabeculoplasty
SPK	superficial punctate keratitis
SRD	serous retinal detachment
TM	trabecular meshwork
TRD	tractional retinal detachment
TSCP	transscleral cyclophotocoagulation
VA	visual acuity
VDRL	Venereal Disease Research Laboratory (test)
WBC	white blood cell

Anatomy and Physiology of the Lids, Eye, Orbit, and Visual System

Charlie Abraham, MD and Thomas E. Bournias, MD

Orbital Anatomy

The orbit is a pear-shaped cavity that forms the eye socket. It is composed of seven bones: frontal, zygoma, maxilla, ethmoid, sphenoid, lacrimal, and palatine (Figure 1-1). Each orbit contains the eyeball, extraocular muscles, fat, and blood vessels. Next to the medial wall, floor, and orbital roof lie the paranasal sinuses, which form an easy route for infection to spread. Pain arising from sinusitis is distributed through these sinuses to different locations of the face.

■ Medial Orbital Wall

The medial orbital wall is composed of four bones, but mainly the ethmoidal bone. The other three bones that form this wall are the maxillary, lacrimal, and the lesser wing of the sphenoid. The lamina papyracea, the thinnest part of the orbit, covers the ethmoid sinuses along the medial wall making this location frequently prone to blowout fractures.

■ Lateral Orbital Wall

The lateral orbital wall is the thickest and strongest wall that protects the posterior half of the eye against trauma. It is formed by two bones: the zygoma and the greater wing of the sphenoid.

■ Orbital Roof

The orbital roof is composed of the frontal bone and the lesser wing of the sphenoid.

■ Orbital Floor

The orbital floor is composed of three bones: maxillary, palatine, and zygomatic. It contains the infraorbital groove and canal where the maxillary branch of the trigeminal nerve (V_2) traverses. The inferior oblique muscle originates from the orbital floor

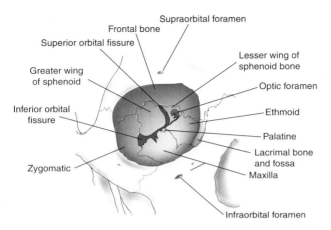

Figure 1-1 • Front view of the bone structure of the right eye. Seven bones make up the bony orbit: 1) frontal, 2) zygoma, 3) sphenoid, 4) maxilla, 5) ethmoid, 6) lacrimal, 7) palatine.

lateral to the opening of the nasolacrimal canal. This muscle is the only extraocular muscle that does not originate from the apex of the orbit.

■ Orbital Apertures

The orbital apex contains the optic foramen, superior orbital fissure, and inferior orbital fissure, which allow passage of the cranial nerves and vessels to and from the orbit. Note that the trochlear nerve (CN IV) and the peripheral divisions of the trigeminal nerve (CN V) lie outside the muscle cone (Figure 1-2).

Optic Foramen

The optic canal extends from the middle cranial fossa to the orbital apex passing through the lesser wing of the sphenoid. The optic nerve, the ophthalmic artery, and sympathetic fibers from the carotid plexus pass through this foramen.

Superior Orbital Fissure

The superior orbital fissure is formed by the greater and lesser wings of the sphenoid. It transmits CNs III and IV, the ophthalmic division of V (includes the lacrimal, frontal, and nasociliary nerve) and VI, and sympathetic nerve fibers. Most of the orbit venous drainage passes through this fissure via the superior ophthalmic vein to the cavernous sinus.

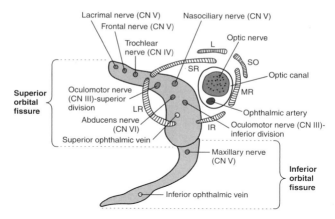

Figure 1-2 • The orbital apex and the superior and inferior orbital fissure. Cranial nerve IV (trochlear) lies outside the muscle cone leaving it unaffected by retrobulbar anesthesia with resultant continued superior oblique function. The orbital apex is the origin of the levator (L), superior oblique (SO), medial rectus (MR), inferior rectus (IR), lateral rectus (LR), and superior rectus (SR).

Inferior Orbital Fissure

The inferior orbital fissure is located between the lateral wall of the orbit and the orbital floor. It is surrounded by the sphenoid, maxillary, and palatine bones. This aperture transmits the infraorbital and zygomatic branches of the maxillary division of cranial nerve V and the inferior ophthalmic vein that leads to the pterygoid plexus. The infraorbital nerve passes through the infraorbital groove in the maxillary bone and exits the infraorbital groove carrying sensation from the lower eyelid, upper lip and teeth, cheek, and gingiva.

Extraocular Muscles (EOMs)

■ Annulus of Zinn

The annulus of Zinn is a fibrous ring formed by the origins of the rectus muscles that encircles the optic foramen. The eye movement is carried out by four rectus and two oblique muscles that act concordantly. Four muscles—the lateral, medial, superior, and inferior recti—originate from the annulus of Zinn; they primarily abduct, adduct, elevate, and depress the globe, respectively (Table 1-1).

■ TABLE 1-1 Extraocular Muscles

Muscle	Origin	Blood Supply	Innervation	Function
Lateral rectus	Annulus of Zinn	Lacrimal artery	VI Abducens	Moves the eye outward
Medial rectus	Annulus of Zinn	Inferior branch of ophthalmic artery	III Oculomotor	Moves the eye inward
Superior rectus	Annulus of Zinn	Superior branch of ophthalmic artery	III Oculomotor	Upward and slightly inward
Inferior rectus	Annulus of Zinn	Inferior branch of ophthalmic artery and infraorbital artery	III Oculomotor	Downward and slightly inward
Superior oblique	Between the annulus of Zinn and periorbita	Superior branch of ophthalmic artery	IV Trochlear	Downward and inward
Inferior oblique	Near orbital rim on the anterior floor of the orbit nasally	Inferior branch of ophthalmic artery and infraorbital artery	III Oculomotor	Upward and outward

Note: The innervation of the extraocular muscles may be remembered by the rhyming mnemonic: L.R. six, S.O. four, all the rest are oculomotor.

Blood Supply of the Orbit

Branches of the external carotid artery contribute a small proportion of the orbital blood supply. However, the main supply is provided by the ophthalmic artery, a branch of the internal carotid artery that travels underneath the optic nerve through the optic canal. The main branches of the ophthalmic artery supply the extraocular muscles, the optic nerve and the retina (central retinal artery), and the anterior segment and the choroid (posterior ciliary arteries). Venous drainage of the orbit is mainly supplied by the superior ophthalmic vein that travels through the superior orbital fissure into the cavernous sinus.

Eyelids

The upper and lower eyelids form a protective covering of the eye against foreign objects and light. The upper eyelid may be raised by the action of the levator muscle innervated by CN III. The orbicularis oculi muscle (CN VII) is its antagonist. Each eyelid contains a tarsal plate that consists of dense connective tissue, not cartilage. Each tarsal plate contains vertically oriented parallel rows of meibomian glands that secrete oil into the tear film via small orifices just posterior to the lashes.

■ Anatomy of the Lacrimal Glands and Excretory System

The lacrimal gland is located in the lacrimal fossa in the superior lateral quadrant of the frontal bone. This gland, along with accessory glands of Krause and Wolfring, produces the serous (aqueous) portion of the tear film. Through the action of the lids, the tear film drains through the punctum in each lid into the canaliculus, then into the lacrimal sac, and finally into the nasolacrimal duct before draining under the inferior turbinate in the nose.

Conjunctiva

The conjunctiva is divided into three areas:
1. Palpebral conjunctiva: the vascular transparent membrane that covers the inner surface of the eyelids
2. Bulbar conjunctiva: the vascular transparent membrane that covers the globe and fuses with Tenon's capsule and attaches to the limbus
3. Fornical conjunctiva: the continuous redundant freely movable part that reflects and attaches to the globe

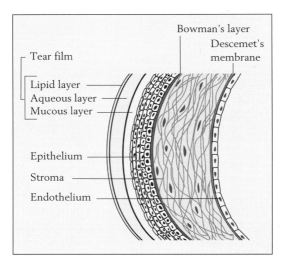

Figure 1-3 • Schematic illustrating the three layers of the precorneal tear film and the five layers of the cornea. *(Reprinted with permission from James B, Chew C, Bron A. Lecture notes on ophthalmology, 9th ed. Oxford: Blackwell Publishing Ltd, 2003.)*

Anatomy of the Eyeball

■ Precorneal Tear Film (Figure 1-3)

The tear film provides an optical surface for the eye in addition to being a main lubricant that nourishes the surface of the cornea with oxygen and other necessary nutrients. It covers the surface of the eyeball (cornea and conjunctiva) and is mainly composed of three layers:

1. The inner layer: mainly formed of mucin secreted by goblet cells within the conjunctiva. Mucin maintains the tear film's adherence to the globe.
2. The intermediate layer: 90% of the tear film and composed of aqueous secreted by the lacrimal and other accessory glands.
3. The outer layer: composed of oil produced by the meibomian glands in the tarsus of the lids. This oily layer prevents premature evaporation of the tear film.

The structures that form the globe (Figure 1-4) are discussed in the following sections.

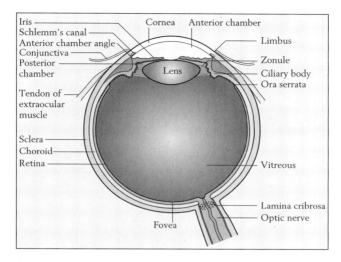

Figure 1-4 • Basic anatomy of the eye. *(Reprinted with permission from James B, Chew C, Bron A. Lecture notes on ophthalmology, 9th ed. Oxford: Blackwell Publishing Ltd, 2003.)*

■ Cornea (Figure 1-3)

The cornea is the transparent "window" in the front of the eye that accounts for two thirds of its refractive power. It consists of five layers:

1. Corneal epithelium: the first layer underneath the tear film, which consists of a five- to seven-cell layer of stratified squamous epithelium. Defects in this epithelium (e.g., abrasion) result in sharp pain because of the rich nerve innervation. However, they may heal quickly (i.e., within 24 hours).
2. Bowman's layer: a very tough layer of collagen fibers between the epithelium and the stroma. This layer is not replaced after injury and may become opacified by scar tissue.
3. Stroma: composes approximately 90%, or 500 µm, of the corneal thickness. It is mainly composed of tiny obliquely and parallel oriented collagen fibers produced by stromal cells (keratocytes). These collagen fibers give the cornea its clarity, strength, and shape.
4. Descemet's membrane: the basement membrane of the corneal endothelium. This membrane is not restored after injury but is replaced by scar tissue.

5. Endothelium: composed of one single layer of cells located posterior to Descemet's membrane. These cells pump fluid to maintain adequate corneal liquid balance thereby maintaining corneal clarity. They rarely mitose and generally decrease in number with age.

■ Sclera

The thin tough white coat of collagen bundles that envelopes the posterior four fifths of the globe. Two potential openings exist in this tissue: an anterior opening for the cornea and a posterior opening for the optic nerve. It is considered to be avascular except for the intrascleral vascular plexus located posterior to the limbus and superficial vessels of the episclera. The sclera is the site of insertion of the extraocular muscles.

■ Limbus

The junction between the cornea and the sclera is called the limbus. Although not a distinct anatomic structure, the limbus is considered important because of its correlation with the chamber angle and because it serves as a surgical landmark. The surgical limbus is about 2 mm wide.

■ Uveal Tract

The uveal tract is the vascular, middle compartment of the eye. It consists of the iris, ciliary body, and choroid. Inflammation of one or more of these components causes uveitis, a condition that requires prompt medical care.

Iris
The iris is the most anterior part of the uveal tract. This structure has a rich blood supply. Involuntary circular (sphincter muscle) and radiating (dilator muscle) fibers control the size of the pupil, which is the opening at the center of the iris. Parasympathetic innervation is the primary mechanism in the sphincter muscle and decreases pupil size (miosis). The dilator muscle is controlled primarily by sympathetic innervation and increases pupil size (mydriasis).

Ciliary Body
The ciliary body is the portion of the uveal tract that lies between the iris and the choroid. It extends from the scleral spur to the end of the retina (ora serrata) and is divided into the anterior pars plicata and the more posterior pars plana. The pars plicata contains about 70 ciliary processes where the aqueous humor is produced. It also consists of the ciliary muscle, which is composed of three layers (mainly under parasympathetic innervation):

longitudinal, radial, and circular. These three groups function as a unit. Sympathetic innervation is thought to play a role in relaxing the muscle. Attached to the ciliary body (in the recesses of the ciliary processes) are small tiny fibers called zonules. These zonules are also attached to the lens capsule at the equator to adjust the lens curvature (its refractive power) to allow adequate focus of light to the back of the eye. This process is called accommodation. Near vision is achieved when the above-mentioned muscles contract, resulting in relaxation of the zonules allowing the lens to become spherical (thereby increasing its refractive power) and focus objects up close. The opposite happens when the muscle fibers relax. With age, the flexibility of the ciliary body muscle and lens gradually deteriorates, leading to difficulty in reading. This condition is called presbyopia, resulting in the need for reading glasses.

Contraction of the longitudinal fibers facilitates the opening of the canal of Schlemm and eventually allows drainage of aqueous humor via the trabecular meshwork.

Choroid

The choroid is the posterior portion of the uveal tract that lies between the retina and sclera. This highly vascular structure provides blood supply to the outer one third of the retina and macula. Blood to the choroid comes from the long and short posterior ciliary arteries as well as from the perforating anterior ciliary arteries. Venous drainage is provided through the four vortex veins passing through the sclera posteriorly. The choroid has a high content of melanocytes, making it a possible site for the development of benign choroidal nevi and malignant choroidal melanoma (the most common intraocular tumor in adults).

■ Lens

The lens is the transparent biconvex structure that lies between the iris and the vitreous humor. The lens is avascular and lacks innervation. It is very rich in protein and consists of an inner nucleus surrounded by an outer cortex. It becomes increasingly cloudy with aging, resulting in cataract formation. The lens is surrounded by a capsule, which is the basement membrane of the lens epithelium.

■ Anterior Chamber

The anterior chamber is defined anteriorly by the cornea and posteriorly by the iris and the pupil. One of the most important landmarks of this chamber is the angle at the junction of the cornea and the iris called the anterior chamber angle. The aqueous humor, produced by the ciliary process of the ciliary body, occupies the anterior chamber. The depth of the anterior chamber is variable. It is deeper in certain conditions, such as aphakia and myopia, and shallower in hyperopia. To assess if the angle is open or narrow, a special lens with mirrors is applied to the surface of the cornea, allowing visualization of the usually unseen angle structures. This procedure is termed gonioscopy (see Figure 2-6). After the aqueous passes through the pupil, it drains out of the eye in the chamber angle via two pathways:

1. The trabecular meshwork (conventional pathway): This route forms the main outflow pathway, accounting for about 85% to 90% of aqueous drainage. Fluid drains through a spongy connective tissue in the anterior chamber angle called the trabecular meshwork. Resistance here is thought to result in primary open-angle glaucoma. The aqueous eventually runs through a tube similar to a lymphatic vessel called Schlemm's canal. Extending from Schlemm's canal, fluid passes through 25 to 30 collector channels, which drain into the deep and midscleral venous plexus.

2. The uveoscleral outflow (nonconventional pathway): This route accounts for about 10% to 15% of aqueous outflow and drains across the ciliary body into the supraciliary space.

■ Posterior Chamber

The posterior chamber is the space between the iris and the lens with its associated zonules.

■ Bruch's Membrane

Bruch's membrane is composed of sheets of connective tissue separating the choriocapillaris of the choroid from the retinal pigment epithelium of the retina. It extends from the optic disc to the anterior peripheral retina called the ora serrata (a structure located between the retina and the pars plana). Defects of Bruch's membrane can be seen in different diseases such as macular degeneration, pseudoxanthoma elasticum, or high myopia.

■ Retina

The retina is the innermost transparent sensory tissue at the back of the eye that develops from the layers of the optic cup. Looking through the ophthalmoscope, the following view of the retina is seen (Figure 1-5). The optic disc is located 20 degrees from the center of the retina, and inside the optic disc is a white circular or oval area called the optic cup. Main retinal blood vessels radiate from the center of the optic nerve. Temporal to the optic nerve, there is a small sensitive central area responsible for central vision called the macula, which is located between the temporal vascular arcades. The macula has two or more retinal ganglion cell layers.

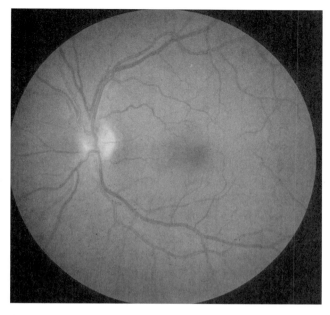

Figure 1-5 • Normal fundus. The macula is located $2^1/_2$ disc diameters temporal and slightly inferior to the optic nerve. The diameter of normal venules is about twice the diameter of the arterioles.

The fovea is a reddish, concave, small depression seen in the center of the macula where vision is most acute.

The retina contains millions of special cells called photoreceptors (rods and cones). The cones are highly concentrated in the fovea and are responsible for central visual acuity and color vision. There are three different types of cones, responding to blue, green, or red light. The rods lie outside the fovea and are responsible for both black and white and night vision. Light rays are captured by these photoreceptors and are converted to electrical impulses. These signals travel through the optic nerve to the brain where they are processed and interpreted as images. The layers of the retina (Figure 1-6) from inside to outside are:

1. **Internal limiting membrane (ILM)**: not a true membrane; formed by footplates of Müller's cells and attachments to the basal lamina
2. **Nerve fiber layer (NFL)**: contains axons of ganglion cells that travel through the optic nerve
3. **Ganglion cell layer (GCL)**: ganglion cell nuclei

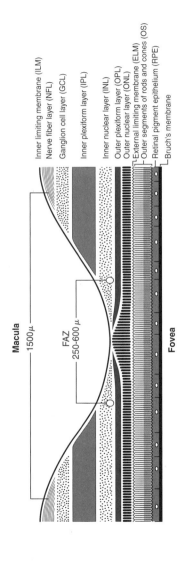

Inner limiting membrane (ILM)
Nerve fiber layer (NFL)
Ganglion cell layer (GCL)
Inner plexiform layer (IPL)
Inner nuclear layer (INL)
Outer plexiform layer (OPL)
Outer nuclear layer (ONL)
External limiting membrane (ELM)
Outer segments of rods and cones (OS)
Retinal pigment epithelium (RPE)
Bruch's membrane

Macula
1500 μ

FAZ
250–600 μ

Fovea

Figure 1-6 • Schematic demonstrating the retina layers. Note that only photoreceptors (and glial and Müller's cells) are present in the fovea. FAZ = foveal avascular zone.

4. **Inner plexiform layer (IPL)**: axons of the bipolar and amacrine cells and dendrites of ganglion cells
5. **Inner nuclear layer (INL)**: nuclei of bipolar, Müller's, horizontal, and amacrine cells
6. **Outer plexiform layer (OPL)**: interconnections between the photoreceptor synaptic bodies and the horizontal and bipolar cells.
7. **Outer nuclear layer (ONL)**: photoreceptor nuclei
8. **External limiting membrane (ELM)**: not a true membrane; attachment site of adjacent photoreceptors and Müller cells
9. **Outer segments (OS)**: layer of rods and cones
10. **Retinal pigment epithelium (RPE)**: monolayer of cells with highly specialized metabolic functions

■ Retinal Blood Vessels

The inner two thirds of the retina is supplied by the retinal blood vessels from the central retinal artery in the optic nerve. A physiologic barrier is achieved due to the tight junctions between the single layer of the endothelial cells of these vessels. These vessels are normally impermeable to tracer substances such as fluorescein. The blood supply of the outer retina and the macula comes from the choroid.

■ Vitreous

The transparent gel that fills four fifths of the eyeball. The vitreous is composed 99% of water. It is adherent to the underlying peripheral retina at the anterior vitreous base (2 mm anterior to the ora serrata) and the posterior vitreous base (4 mm posterior to the ora serrata). Additional attachments also exist at the disc margin, the perifoveal region, and the posterior lens capsule. However, with age, the vitreous may spontaneously separate from the retina (vitreous detachment). This is the most common inciting event associated with a rhegmatogenous retinal detachment.

Optic Nerve and Visual Pathways

Axons of the retinal ganglion cells travel to each optic nerve. From here they travel to the optic chiasm where the nasal fibers partially decussate and travel through the contralateral optic tract and synapse at the contralateral lateral geniculate nucleus (LGN). The temporal fibers continue through the ipsilateral optic tract and synapse at their ipsilateral LGN. Fibers then radiate from the lateral geniculate body via the optic radiation to the visual cortex of the occipital lobe in the brain. The fibers of the optic radiation leave the LGN and travel around the temporal

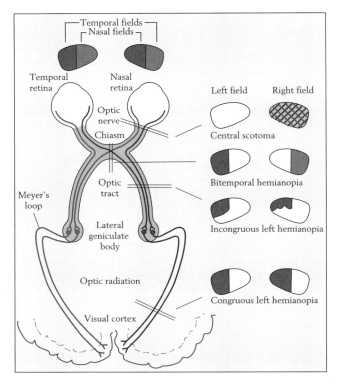

Figure 1-7 • Anatomy of the visual pathway with associated field defects resulting from lesions at various sites. *(Reprinted with permission from James B, Chew C, Bron A. Lecture notes on ophthalmology, 9th ed. Oxford: Blackwell Publishing Ltd, 2003.)*

horn of the lateral ventricle, approaching the anterior tip of the temporal lobe (Meyer's loop). They then sweep posteriorly toward the visual area of the occipital lobe. Macular function represents approximately 90% of the visual cortex. Lesions along various locations of the visual pathway result in various and characteristic field defects (Figure 1-7).

2 Basic Ophthalmic Examination

Charlie Abraham, MD, Preeya Kshettry,
and Thomas E. Bournias, MD

History

The purpose of the history is to assess visual function and ocular health. The physician should elicit the chief complaint and history of present illness. Then he or she should ask questions about past ocular history, such as eye injuries, diseases, or surgeries. Next, the physician should obtain information about ocular and systemic medications, as well as relevant past medical history such as diabetes mellitus and hypertension, because they often have ocular sequelae. Any family history of ocular and systemic diseases, such as glaucoma, age-related macular degeneration (AMD), diabetes, or hypertension, should be noted because patients have increased risk of developing these diseases if other family members are affected.

Ophthalmic Examination

A basic ophthalmic examination includes investigation of anatomic structures and testing of the physiologic function of the eye and visual system.

■ Visual Acuity

Visual acuity (VA) refers to the ability of the eye to identify images at a certain distance, usually 20 feet. VA is represented by a fraction. The denominator refers to what a normal healthy eye can see in comparison to the numerator, which represents what the tested eye can see. Therefore, a VA of 20/40 means that what a normal eye sees at 40 feet, the tested eye can see at 20 feet.

Although a variety of methods may be used to assess VA, a Snellen chart is typically used in ophthalmology clinics. Each eye should be tested individually; therefore, it is necessary to cover one eye while testing the other. VA should be first tested while the patient is wearing his or her corrective lenses (VA_{CC}) and reassessed without correction (VA_{SC}).

A VA below normal (less than 20/20 on a Snellen chart) can be due to either a refractive error or to a disease process in the eye. Usual refractive errors are myopia, hyperopia, and astigmatism. Myopia (nearsightedness) results when the eye is too long or the cornea is very steep forming an image in front of the retina requiring concave lenses for correction (Figures 2-1 and 2-2). Hyperopia (farsightedness) results when the eye is too short or the cornea is too flat forming an image behind the retina necessitating convex lenses for correction (see Figures 2-1 and 2-2). Astigmatism results when the cornea or lens has a different refracting power in one meridian than another (e.g., the shape of a football). The pinhole test is often used to differentiate between a refractive error and pathology.

Pinhole Test

If VA is below normal, the patient is asked to read the eye chart by looking through a pinhole occluder. A pinhole allows only central rays of light into the eye so that the refractive surfaces of the eye are not used to assess VA in this case. If there is an underlying refractive error, the patient should improve by at least one to two lines. If no improvement was noted with the pinhole, refractive error is less likely to be the cause of reduced vision. Examination may then disclose the cause of the decreased vision.

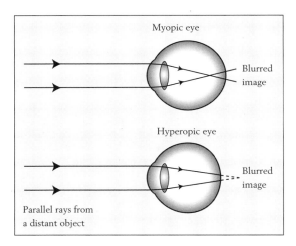

Figure 2-1 • Diagram of myopia and hyperopia. In myopia the optical power of the eye is too high and the image falls in front of the retina. In hyperopia the optical power of the eye is too low and the image forms behind the retina. *(Reprinted with permission from James B, Chew C, Bron A. Lecture notes on ophthalmology, 9th ed. Oxford: Blackwell Publishing Ltd, 2003.)*

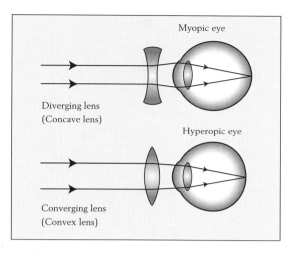

Figure 2-2 • Correction of ametropia with proper spectacle lenses. Concave lenses correct myopia; convex lenses correct hyperopia. *(Reprinted with permission from James B, Chew C, Bron A.* Lecture notes on ophthalmology, *9th ed. Oxford: Blackwell Publishing Ltd, 2003.)*

Near Visual Acuity

Near vision refers to the ability of the eye to see clearly at a normal reading distance. Corrective lenses should be used if needed. The patient is asked to read a handheld card placed about 14 inches away. Causes for decreased near acuity can be central cataracts or presbyopia. Presbyopia affects most people soon after the age of 40 years. The lens loses its ability to accommodate (focus at near) with age, resulting in the need for reading glasses or bifocals after the age of 40 years (see Chapter 1, Ciliary Body, p. 9).

■ External Examination

The periocular tissues and lids should be examined with attention to the presence of ectropion (outward turning of the eyelid margin), entropion (inward turning of the eyelid margin), and blepharoptosis (drooping of the eyelid).

■ Extraocular Muscles

Extraocular muscle (EOM) motility should be assessed in six cardinal positions of gaze (Figure 2-3). In each of these cardinal positions,

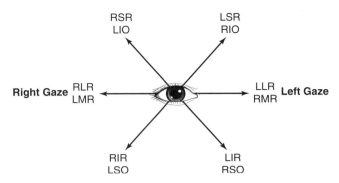

Figure 2-3 • Cardinal positions of gaze of the right eye with the corresponding yoke muscle in the left eye. LR, Lateral rectus; MR, medial rectus; SR, superior rectus; IR, inferior rectus; IO, inferior oblique; SO, superior oblique.

one muscle of each eye is the prime mover. Each EOM in one eye has a yoke muscle in the other eye. The examiner holds a finger about 10 to 14 inches in front of the patient and asks the patient to watch the finger as it moves into the cardinal positions, as if drawing the letter H. It is important that the patient maintain fixation on the finger without moving his or her head. If there is a restriction, it is possible to identify an isolated weakness or paralysis of an EOM.

▒ Confrontational Visual Field Test

The confrontational visual field (CVF) test is used as a screening tool for prominent visual field abnormalities. Essentially the examiner compares his or her own gross visual field function (assumed to be normal) with that of the patient. The examiner sits about 3 feet in front of the patient and asks the patient to cover one eye. Covering the opposite eye, the examiner presents a varied number of fingers to the patient in all four quadrants and compares the patient's response to the number presented. The test is repeated for the opposite eye.

▒ Pupil Examination

Observe the pupil size, shape, and reaction to light. Upon shining a light in one eye, the examiner should normally observe constriction of both pupils equally.
• **Direct reflex:** pupil constriction in the illuminated eye.
• **Consensual reflex:** pupil constriction in the nonilluminated eye.

- **Swinging flashlight test:** compares the consensual and direct reflexes obtained by shining a brisk light on each eye alternately and observing the pupillary response (see pupil, Chapter 6).
- **Relative afferent pupillary defect (RAPD):** if an RAPD is present, one sees a stronger consensual reflex than direct reflex (see pupil, Chapter 6).

■ Slit Lamp Examination (Biomicroscopy)

The slit lamp is used to examine various depths of tissues (e.g., cornea) or spaces (e.g., anterior chamber) for pathologic processes by using narrow beams of light and retroillumination.

Eyelids

Lashes should be inspected for signs of blepharitis or trichiasis (lash turning in and rubbing against the eye). Meibomian gland orifices should be examined behind the lashes. Their position, size, and presence of obstruction/secretions should be noted.

Conjunctiva

Both bulbar (conjunctiva on the globe) and palpebral conjunctiva (conjunctiva lining internal aspects of the lids) should be examined for blood vessel congestion/erythema or foreign bodies.

Cornea

Inspect for deposits or defects on the cornea, thinning of its surface, or cloudiness, as well as the presence of blood vessels invading its surface. Evaluate the quantity and quality of the tear film. A normal amount of tear film should leave a 1-mm meniscus between the globe and the edge of the lower lid. Then check the tear break-up time (quality of the outer oily layer to prevent evaporation).

Anterior Chamber

Look for white blood cells floating in the aqueous humor, representing iritis. This can be seen by focusing a thin oblique beam on the anterior chamber and noting passing cells (such as dust particles visible in the projector light path in a movie theater). Also look for flare (scattering of the slit lamp beam), which indicates leakage of proteins into the anterior chamber. Cells and flare are indicative of anterior chamber reaction due to inflammation such as that seen in uveitis (Plate 1). The presence of pigmented cells may be seen, indicating pigment dispersion syndrome or a possible retinal detachment. Evaluate the clarity of the aqueous humor and assess the depth of the anterior chamber.

Iris

Inspect iris color as well as the presence of nevi or posterior synechiae (adhesion of the iris to the lens capsule). Also look for growth of blood vessels on the surface of the iris (rubeosis iridis), which may occur in diabetics or other conditions causing occlusive vascular disease.

Lens

Carefully look for opacities, which may represent cataract formation.

■ Intraocular Pressure

Goldmann applanation tonometry is widely used by ophthalmologists as a standard technique for measuring intraocular pressure (IOP). After anesthetizing the eye with a fluorescein-containing anesthetic drop, using the cobalt blue light setting on the slit lamp, the physician presses the tip of the tonometer against the cornea. The pressure is then determined by measuring the amount of aqueous displaced. The thickness of the cornea may alter the IOP reading. Thicker corneas read falsely higher than the true IOP and thinner corneas read falsely lower than the true IOP. The average corneal thickness is 545 μm. Every additional 20 μm of thickness implies that the true IOP is actually about 1 mm Hg lower than the IOP reading. The opposite holds for thinner corneas. IOP can also be assessed using a Tono-Pen (Automated Ophthalmics),which is not altered appreciably by variation in corneal thickness.

■ Fundus Examination

With dilation the entire fundus up to the ora serrata may be visualized. The physician should inspect the macula, vessels, optic nerve, and peripheral retina (see Figure 1-5).

Macula

Examine the macula closely for signs of drusen or microaneurysms. Inspect for pigment change or membranes, as well as the presence of a good foveal reflex.

Blood Vessels

Describe the appearance of the blood vessels and note their caliber looking for signs of attenuation. Normally the venules/arteriole diameter is about 3:2. Check for arteriovenous nicking (AVN) as seen in hypertensive retinopathy.

Optic Nerve

Determine that the disc margins are sharp. Inspect for swelling or hemorrhage. The neuroretinal rim should be orange-pink.

Assessment of the nerve fiber layer is crucial to diagnose and monitor progression in glaucoma. Note the cup/disc (C/D) ratio and overall position of the cup within the optic nerve.

Peripheral Retina

Evaluate the peripheral retina with scleral depression for breaks, tears, or lattice degeneration (thinning of the peripheral retina).

Vitreous Humor

Look for vitreous hemorrhage or detachment (Plate 18). Some patients describe opacities in the vitreous as "floating spots." The majority of these floaters are due to a benign process that is often seen in elderly and highly myopic patients. Hemorrhage may be seen with proliferative diabetic retinopathy or with a retinal tear. Pigmented cells in the vitreous (Plate 2) may indicate the presence of a retinal tear.

Other Examinations and Testing

■ Amsler Grid

The Amsler grid (Figure 2-4) is a tool for detection of abnormalities in central vision. It is frequently used to investigate macular disorders such as AMD. In this test, the central 10 to 20 degrees of the visual field in each eye is assessed individually. The patient is asked to cover one eye and to fixate on a central dot while simultaneously looking at the grid to see if the grid lines are parallel and complete. The presence of distortion or missing lines may indicate macular dysfunction.

■ A-Scan Ultrasonography (Biometry)

High-frequency sound waves are used to measure axial length as well as to study structures of the eye that are not directly visible. Sound beams are aimed in a straight line, and recorded echoes are correlated with structures in the eye.

■ Automated Perimetry (Static Perimetry)

Automated perimetry is performed with an instrument that uses fixed light locations to test for visual field defects. Automated perimetry is more useful for detecting smaller defects than kinetic perimetry. It functions by facilitating statistical comparisons between the patient and a normal subject. This modality is usually used to monitor for the presence or progression of glaucoma.

■ B-Scan Ultrasonography

B-scan ultrasonography provides a two-dimensional (cross-sectional) image of the eye from posterior to the iris to just

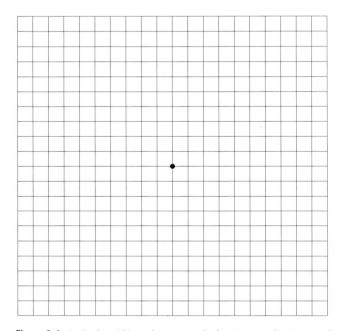

Figure 2-4 • An Amsler grid is used to test macular function or to detect a central or paracentral scotoma.

posterior to the globe. It is an excellent modality for defining ocular anatomy when visualization in the eye is obstructed by media opacities. This modality may be used to identify intraocular foreign bodies, tumors/masses, or retinal/choroidal detachments.

■ Cover-Uncover Test

The cover-uncover test is used to determine the presence and direction of deviations from the normal ocular axes (strabismus). Essentially, the ability of both eyes to focus simultaneously on the same object is tested. The patient is asked to look at a distant target using both eyes. Covering one eye, the observer watches the movement of the noncovered eye. The same is repeated for the opposite eye. Inward movement of the noncovered eye is known as exotropia (if the nonoccluded eye turns in to fixate, it has an outward deviation). Esotropia is present when the nonoccluded eye turns outward.

■ Cross-Cover Testing

Cross-cover testing is done to determine the degree of misalignment between the eyes. While alternately covering each eye, the examiner places prisms in front of one eye to neutralize the visual axis deviation, if present. The correct diopter prism needed to neutralize the deviation is determined when movement of the eye, while alternating the covering of each eye, no longer occurs. The degree of dissociation between the two eyes is equal to the power of the prism placed in front of the eye. (The tip of the prism is held in the direction of the deviation.)

■ Fluorescein Angiography

By injecting fluorescein (yellow) or indocyanine (green) dyes into the venous blood system, fluorescein angiography is used to study blood circulation of the retina and the underlying choroid. Sets of consecutive pictures are taken by a special camera to view the blood distribution in the retinal/choroidal vessels. Dye may leak from abnormal vessels (e.g., diabetic retinopathy or choroidal neovascularization in macular degeneration) or may fail to demonstrate normal passage through arterioles due to retinal capillary closure, indicating ischemia (e.g., branch retinal vein occlusion; Figure 2-5).

■ Frequency-Doubling Perimetry

Frequency-doubling perimetry is performed to assess early visual field loss. Although controversial, it is thought that the frequency-doubling illusion phenomenon may isolate a specific subtype of retinal ganglion cells thought to be targeted in early glaucoma. This may result in the detection of visual field change sooner than standard perimetry.

■ GDx

GDx refers to a scanning laser polarimeter that quantitatively measures the thickness of the retinal nerve fiber layer (RNFL). This device may assist in following progression of glaucoma by detecting any loss of the RNFL by measuring the retardation of a laser beam passing through the birefringent fibers of the RNFL.

■ Goldmann Perimetry (Kinetic Perimetry)

Goldmann perimetry is used to map visual fields. A target is projected into a dome as the examiner observes patient fixation on a central point. The size and intensity of the target can be altered to assess visual fields. The target is moved from the periphery of the dome toward the central fixation point, and the patient upon

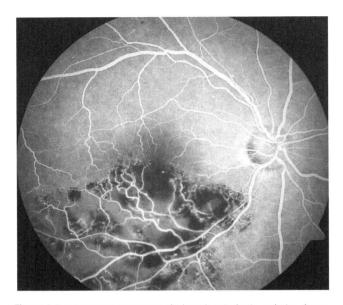

Figure 2-5 • Fluorescein angiogram of a branch retinal vein occlusion demonstrating capillary nonperfusion (black areas).

seeing the target can press a buzzer connected to the machine. This test is used most frequently in neurologic testing.

■ Gonioscopy

Gonioscopy is a technique whereby a handheld lens with mirrors is placed against the anesthetized cornea so that the normally unseen anterior angle structures may be visualized. The degree to which the angle is open is evaluated as are signs of pathologic processes, such as peripheral anterior synechia as may be seen in narrow angles and inflammatory disorders (Figure 2-6).

■ Heidelberg Retinal Tomography

Heidelberg retinal tomography (HRT) captures a three-dimensional image of the posterior pole of the eye. It is mainly used to picture and monitor the optic nerve in glaucoma. HRT provides high-definition images of both diffuse and focal defects in the retinal nerve fiber layer.

■ Keratometry

Keratometry is used to assess corneal curvature and the presence of an aspherical ocular surface (astigmatism). This test is important

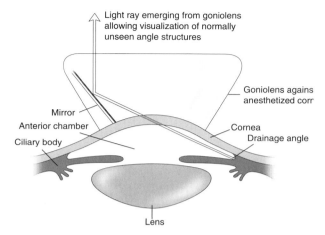

Figure 2-6 • Indirect gonioscopy. A gonioscopy lens with specialized mirrors is placed against the anesthetized cornea so that the normally unseen angle structures may be identified at the slit lamp.

for calculating the power needed of an artificial intraocular lens implant, contact lens fitting, and refractive surgery.

■ Optical Coherence Tomography

As a new noninvasive technique, optical coherence tomography (OCT) is used to image the retina and its layers, as well as to assess the retinal nerve fiber layer thickness. In this respect, OCT can be used to evaluate retinal and macular diseases, as well as to monitor glaucomatous loss of the nerve fibers.

■ Pachymetry

Pachymetry is a test used to measure corneal thickness. The central corneal thickness (CCT) is measured to determine if patients may undergo refractive procedures such as laser-assisted in situ keratomileusis (LASIK). Recently, CCT has been used to assist in determining what the relative risk of a patient with ocular hypertension has of developing glaucomatous optic nerve or visual field changes.

■ Specular Microscopy

In this modality, highly magnified pictures of the endothelial cells lining the posterior aspect of the cornea are obtained by use of a special microscope. The quality, as well as the number of endothelial cells, is inspected. Corneas with a decreased number of endothelial cells are at increased risk of corneal decompensation (edema/clouding), especially if the eye undergoes surgery (e.g., cataract surgery).

■ Stereo Disc Photography

A retinal camera is used to take three-dimensional photographs of the optic disc. This technique is useful in glaucoma management for monitoring changes in the disc over time.

3 Differential Diagnosis of Ocular Complaints

Jerry Lai, MD and Thomas E. Bournias, MD

Red Eye

■ Differential Diagnosis

- Conjunctivitis (see p. 83)
- Dry eye (see p. 81)
- Blepharitis (see p. 79)
- Subconjunctival hemorrhage (see p. 84 and Plate 10)
- Inflamed pinguecula/pterygium (see p. 86 and Figure 7-1)
- Episcleritis (see p. 88)
- Scleritis (see p. 89 and Plate 12)
- Acute angle-closure glaucoma (ACG) (see p. 118)
- Anterior uveitis (see p. 121 and Plate 1)
- Corneal abrasion (see p. 35), corneal foreign body, or corneal infiltrate/ulcer (see pp. 99–100 and Plate 3)
- Conjunctival tumor: e.g., hemorrhagic lymphoma, which is a pink, smooth, elevated, subepithelial mass that may be bright red when hemorrhagic. It is rare, but seen more commonly with systemic lymphoma or immunosuppression.
- Allergic reaction: abrupt or gradual onset of hyperemia with associated itching and burning. Conjunctival edema and watery or mucoid discharge are seen on slit lamp examination.

   See Table 3-1 to differentiate clinical manifestations of common causes of red eye.

■ Initial Follow-up/Management

- Follow-up with an ophthalmologist within 24 hours
- Immediate examination with ophthalmologist if associated with loss of vision, significant eye pain, or contact lens use

Eye Pain: Superficial (Including Foreign Body Sensation)

■ Differential Diagnosis

- Dry eye syndrome (see p. 81)
- Blepharitis (see p. 79)
- Conjunctivitis (see p. 83)

■ TABLE 3-1 Clinical Manifestations of Common Disorders Causing Red Eye

Clinical Manifestation	Bacterial Conjunctivitis	Viral Conjunctivitis	Allergic Conjunctivitis	Acute Iritis	Acute Angle-Closure Glaucoma	Corneal Infiltrate
Pain	N	N	N	Y	Y	Y
Blurred vision	N	N	N	Y	Y	Y
Photophobia	N	N	N	Y	Y	Y
Colored halos	N	N	N	N	Y	N
Itching	N	N	Y	N	N	N
Discharge	Thick	Watery	Watery/mucoid			Thin-thick
Conjunctival hyperemia	Y	Y	Y	Y	Y	Y
Ciliary flush	N	N	N	Y	Y	Y
Corneal opacification	N	Y/N	N	N	Y	Y
Shallow anterior chamber	N	N	N	N	Y	N
Pupillary abnormality	N	N	N	Constricted	Mid-dilated	N
Elevated intraocular pressure	N	N	N	Y/N	Y	N
Enlarged preauricular node	N	Y	N	N	N	N

Y, Manifestation typically present; N, manifestation typically not present.

- Episcleritis (see p. 88 and Plate 12)
- Inflamed pinguecula/pterygium (see p. 86 and Figure 7-1)
- Foreign body (corneal or conjunctival) (see p. 37)
- Corneal disorder including abrasion (see p. 35), superficial punctate keratitis, infiltrate/ulcer (see pp. 99–100 and Plate 3), recurrent corneal erosion (see p. 92)
- Contact lens–related problem (see p. 98)
- Trichiasis: inwardly directed eyelash rubbing against the cornea presenting with a foreign body sensation, irritation, and epiphora (tearing). Scarring and inflammation may be seen along the eyelid. In severe cases, corneal ulceration may occur.
- Entropion: inward rotation of the tarsus (eyelid) presenting with foreign body sensation, irritation, epiphora/discharge, and secondary blepharospasm. Eventually, conjunctival metaplasia and corneal scarring may occur.
- Ectropion: outward rotation of the tarsus presenting with symptoms related to corneal and conjunctival exposure, including foreign body sensation, burning, epiphora, decreased vision, and photophobia. Eventually, conjunctival keratinization and corneal ulceration may occur.

■ Initial Follow-up/Management

- Topical anesthesia
- Immediate examination if history of trauma, contact lens use, poor relief from topical anesthesia, or associated with loss of vision or significant eye pain (such as inability to keep eyes open)

Eye Pain: Deep, Severe

■ Differential Diagnosis

- Anterior uveitis (see p. 121 and Plate 1)
- Scleritis (see p. 89 and Plate 12)
- Corneal ulcer (see pp. 99–100 and Plate 3)
- Acute angle-closure glaucoma (ACG) (see p. 118)
- Ocular ischemic syndrome: chronic arterial hypoperfusion presenting with visual loss and ocular angina (dull ache over eye or brow). Examination findings may include neovascularization of the iris or posterior segment, iritis, retinal arteriolar narrowing and pulsation, retinal venous dilation, retinal hemorrhages and microaneurysms, and occasionally a cherry-red spot.

■ Initial Follow-up/Management

- Immediate ophthalmologic consultation particularly with any change in vision or pupillary response

Eye Pain: Orbital/Periocular

■ Differential Diagnosis

- Sinusitis: presents with bilateral (or unilateral), frontal or retro-orbital headache or pressure often associated with nasal discharge
- Orbital pseudotumor: acute, nongranulomatous inflammatory disease presenting with abrupt pain, conjunctival injection or swelling, eyelid edema, exophthalmos, and motility restriction
- Optic neuritis (see p. 72)
- Diabetic cranial nerve palsy (see p. 148)
- Ocular ischemic syndrome (see Eye Pain: Deep, Severe, p. 29)
- Acute angle-closure glaucoma (ACG) (see p. 118)
- Anterior uveitis (see p. 121 and Plate 1)
- Herpes zoster ophthalmicus (see p. 96)

■ Initial Follow-up/Management

- Evaluation by ophthalmologist within a few hours (immediately if associated with loss of vision)

Vision Loss: Sudden, Painless

■ Differential Diagnosis

- Optic neuritis: sometimes associated with pain (see p. 72)
- Ischemic optic neuropathy (see pp. 75–78)
- Retinal vessel occlusion (CRAO/BRAO or CRVO/BRVO) (see pp. 127–133 and Plates 15 and 16)
- Retinal detachment (RD) (see p. 136 and Plate 19)
- Vitreous hemorrhage (see p. 135)
- Exudative or hemorrhagic age-related macular degeneration (AMD) (see p. 139 and Plate 21)

■ Initial Follow-up/Management

- Immediate ophthalmologic consultation

Vision Loss: Sudden, Painful

■ Differential Diagnosis

- Corneal ulcer (see p. 99 and Plate 3)
- Acute ACG (see p. 118)
- Optic neuritis: often painless (see p. 72)
- Uveitis (see Chapter 9 and Plate 1)
- Acute hydrops (in keratoconus): rupture of Descemet's membrane resulting in stromal overhydration presenting as unilateral red, painful eye with photophobia. On slit lamp examination,

corneal edema is seen. Corneal ulceration must be ruled out as it has a similar presentation.

- Ocular ischemic syndrome (see Eye Pain: Deep, Severe, p. 29)
- Endophthalmitis (see p. 123)
- Keratitis: corneal inflammation usually caused by an infectious agent associated with conjunctival inflammation, lid edema, discharge, anterior chamber reaction, and, occasionally, hypopyon
- Migraine: unilateral, throbbing headache associated with nausea, fatigue, and photophobia. Visual field defects, blurry vision, and scintillating flashes may precede or follow the headache.

■ Initial Follow-up/Management

- Immediate ophthalmologic consultation

Vision Loss: Gradual, Painless (over Weeks to Years)

■ Differential Diagnosis

- Cataract (see p. 106)
- Refractive error: uncorrected myopia, hyperopia, and astigmatism may result in blurred vision
- Open-angle glaucoma (see pp. 101–109)
- Diabetic retinopathy (see pp. 145–148 and Plates 22 and 23)
- Nonexudative macular degeneration (see p. 139 and Plate 20)

■ Initial Follow-up/Management

- Not emergent: ophthalmologic consultation in 24 to 48 hours

Vision Loss: Transient

■ Differential Diagnosis

- Papilledema (see p. 70 and Plate 7)
- Amaurosis fugax: unilateral ophthalmic artery insufficiency caused by emboli or vasospasm lasting seconds to hours. Dilated fundus examination may reveal cholesterol emboli (Hollenhorst plaque) in arterial bifurcations.
- Migraine (see Vision Loss: Sudden, Painful, p. 31)
- Vertebrobasilar arterial insufficiency: transient bilateral blurred vision lasting seconds to minutes. Sometimes associated with flashes and other neurologic symptoms, including vertigo and syncope.
- Corneal or tear film abnormality: vision usually improves with blinking as ocular surface debris are brushed away.
- Ischemic optic neuropathy (see pp. 75–78)

- Ocular ischemic syndrome (see Eye Pain: Deep, Severe, p. 29)
- Impending central retinal vein occlusion (CRVO) (see p. 130)
- Sudden change in blood pressure: transient, bilateral, blurred vision lasting seconds to minutes often associated with flashes and light-headedness

■ Initial Follow-up/Management
- Immediate examination by physician if associated with other neurologic complaints
- Examination with ophthalmologist within 24 hours

Distortion of Vision

■ Differential Diagnosis
- Migraine (see Vision Loss: Sudden, Painful, p. 31)
- Cataract (see p. 166)
- Corneal irregularity: an irregularity of focus caused by any of a variety of corneal erosions, dysplasias, dystrophies, or degenerations differentiated by their appearance on slit lamp examination. Refractive surface or index changes may result in distortion or monocular diplopia.
- Refractive error: blurred vision caused by aberrant focus of image on the retina. May cause headaches with prolonged reading. May also present as monocular diplopia.
- AMD (see p. 139) or other macular disease (e.g., epiretinal membrane). An epiretinal membrane is an avascular, fibrocellular, proliferative membrane on the inner surface of the retina presenting with central vision loss with or without metamorphopsia.
- Retinal detachment (RD) (see p. 136 and Plate 19)

■ Initial Follow-up/Management
- Immediate examination with ophthalmologist if visual distortion is sudden in onset (especially if associated with decreased central vision)
- Examination within 24 hours if central vision intact

Floaters/Flashes

■ Differential Diagnosis
- Posterior vitreous detachment (PVD) (see p. 133)
- Vitreous floaters/condensation or vitreous hemorrhage (see pp. 133–136 and Plate 18)
- Retinal tear or detachment (see p. 136)
- Migraine (see Vision Loss: Sudden, Painful, p. 31)

- Rapid eye movements: transient single flash most common in a dark room
- Posterior uveitis (see p. 123)
- Retinitis: infections or inflammatory (e.g., cytomegalovirus retinitis) (see pp. 162–163 and Plate 24)

■ Initial Follow-up/Management

- Examination with ophthalmologist within 24 hours with dilated fundus examination
- Immediate examination if associated with loss of central vision

Double Vision (Diplopia): Monocular

Diplopia persists when the unaffected eye is occluded.

■ Differential Diagnosis

- Tear film irregularity (see pp. 79–83) or refractive error
- Corneal opacity or irregularity (e.g., keratoconus)
- Cataract: most common with cortical cataract (see p. 166)
- Dislocated lens: disruption of lens zonule fibers from trauma presenting with diplopia, visual distortion, or blurred vision
- Retinal detachment (RD) (see p. 136 and Plate 19)
- Macular disease, including AMD, RD, central serous chorioretinopathy, epiretinal membrane (ERM), macular edema

■ Initial Follow-up/Management

- Follow-up with ophthalmologist within 24 to 48 hours
- Immediate examination if acute (rarely acute in monocular diplopia)

Double Vision (Diplopia): Binocular

Diplopia resolves when either eye is covered.

■ Differential Diagnosis

- Decompensation of existing phoria: Intermittent diplopia that may worsen with certain eye movements. A phoria may be detected by the cover-uncover test (see p. 22).
- Myasthenia gravis: defective acetylcholine synaptic transmission that may result in intermittent diplopia and bilateral, asymmetric ptosis that worsens throughout the day and can be elicited through fatigue. Administration of edrophonium chloride dose causes immediate, temporary relief of symptoms.
- Cranial nerve (CN III, IV, or VI) palsy: paresis associated with constant diplopia that worsens with gaze away from the

deviation. Etiologic factors include tumor, aneurysm, trauma, and infarct.

- CN III: vertical and/or horizontal diplopia with the affected eye deviating in an inferolateral direction. May be associated with ptosis and a fixed, dilated pupil.
- CN IV: vertical diplopia with the affected eye deviating superiorly. The patient may compensate with a head tilt.
- CN VI: horizontal diplopia with affected eye deviating medially.

- Mechanical restriction (e.g., thyroid eye disease[see p. 151], tumor, orbital pseudotumor, orbital wall fracture) (see p. 45)
- Central nervous system lesion [internuclear ophthalmoplegia (INO), vertebrobasilar insufficiency]: An INO is an injury to the medial longitudinal fasciculus (often seen in multiple sclerosis) presenting with deficient adduction of the ipsilateral eye (see p. 149).

▧ Initial Follow-up/Management

- Examination with an ophthalmologist if acute within 24 hours
- Immediate examination with ophthalmologist if acute, post-surgical, or traumatic
- Immediate examination with neurologist if associated with other neurologic complaints

Ocular Trauma

Charlie Abraham, MD, Preeya Kshettry, and
Thomas E. Bournias, MD

Corneal Abrasion

Injuries directed to the surface of the cornea may result in scratches or abrasions of the epithelium. The epithelium is torn from its attachment at the basement membrane. Usually there is a great amount of associated pain because the cornea is highly innervated.

■ History

- Acute sharp pain, occasionally with movement of extraocular muscles
- Tearing, redness, and foreign body (FB) sensation
- Light sensitivity (photophobia) with or without blepharospasm (twitching of the eyelid)
- Blurred vision
- History of scratching/trauma to the eye

■ Clinical Manifestations

- Localized irregular corneal epithelial defect that stains with fluorescein dye
- Conjunctival injection
- Occasionally, intra- and subepithelial lines may be seen representing poor adhesion between the epithelium and Bowman's membrane
- Occasionally, an associated iritis

■ Differential Diagnosis

- Corneal FB: slit lamp examination may reveal an FB on the ocular surface or under an eyelid
- Corneal ulcer/infiltrate (Plate 3): usually seen as a focal opacity in the corneal stroma on slit lamp examination
- Herpes simplex keratitis (Figure 4-1): usually unilateral and sometimes associated with a vesicular skin rash and follicular conjunctivitis

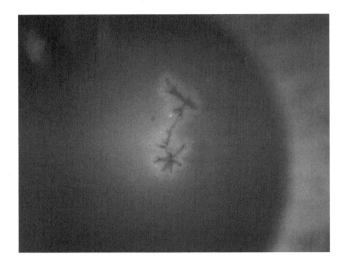

Figure 4-1 • Typical dendritic ulcer seen in herpes simplex keratitis.

- Recurrent corneal erosion: recurring episodes of intermittent, sudden pain often upon awakening. Slit lamp examination may reveal minimal to no evidence of epithelial defect/staining. Diagnosis is often by history.

■ Diagnostic Evaluation

- Slit lamp examination using fluorescein to evaluate the size of the abrasion and its location
- Eversion of the eyelids to look for FBs

■ Treatment

Corneal epithelium has the ability to expand and fill in the defect (often within 24 hours if not too large). As clinically observed, superficial corneal abrasions normally take 1 to 2 days to heal. However, deep abrasions are more likely to leave a permanent scar and should be managed and monitored more aggressively.

- Artificial tears/ointments for smaller abrasions.
- Cycloplegic agent (cyclopentolate 1% or homatropine, one drop 2 to 4 times per day) if an associated iritis is present.
- Topical broad spectrum antibiotic (e.g., tobramycin, gatifloxacin, or moxifloxacin, one drop four times per day)

with larger abrasions or contact lens wearers (contact lens wearers need *Pseudomonas* coverage).

- Ointments blur vision more than drops but offer a better barrier between the abrasion and eyelid.
- Nonsteroidal anti-inflammatory drops (NSAID) (e.g., ketorolac tromethamine 0.4%, one drop four times per day) for pain. Avoid steroid drops because they may retard epithelial healing.
- Bandage soft contact lens may also be effective.
- Reserve patching for only severe cases and do not use if patient wears contact lenses or achieved injury with organic matter (e.g., tree branch).
- Consider debriding loose epithelium because it may inhibit healing.
- No contact lens use (except bandage contact lens under physician's care) until completely healed.

■ Follow-up

- Peripheral or small abrasions usually require follow-up in 2 to 5 days.
- Deep, large, or central abrasions require next-day follow-up. If improvement is noted the following day, the patient may return in 2 to 5 days.
- Careful attention should be paid when:
  - Complicated with infection
  - Missed FB
  - Pain persists for more than 24 hours
- Contact lens wearers should be seen daily and treated with topical antibiotics (e.g., tobramycin, moxifloxacin, gatifloxacin 4 to 8 times per day) until resolution.

Corneal and Conjunctival Foreign Body

Corneal and conjunctival foreign bodies (FBs) are usually related to ocular trauma. Objects traveling at high speeds can be embedded in the cornea or conjunctiva, causing visual problems. The prognosis is good when the FB can be removed easily. However, in the cornea if a rust ring is seen around the object or if scarring develops, the visual prognosis is slightly worse. There is also a risk of infection, tissue necrosis, and penetrating globe injuries with corneal and conjunctival FBs.

■ History

- FB sensation, tearing, and photophobia
- Blurred vision
- History of trauma to the eye

■ Clinical Manifestations

- Presence of foreign matter on the surface or embedded in the cornea or conjunctiva
- Corneal stromal infiltrate if the FB has been present for more than 24 hours
- Rust ring in cornea if FB contains iron
- Conjunctival injection and lid edema (FB may be lodged under lid)
- Superficial punctate keratitis (SPK)
- Mild anterior chamber (AC) reaction: cell/flare

■ Differential Diagnosis

- Corneal abrasion: usually there is an epithelial defect that stains with fluorescein on slit lamp examination and no FB is detected.
- Keratitis: general signs of inflammation of the cornea may be present. No rust ring is seen on the corneal surface.
- Dry eye: patient complains of FB sensation. No history of trauma and no FB found. Slit lamp examination reveals decreased tear film and SPK.

■ Diagnostic Evaluation

- Check visual acuity (if difficult secondary to blepharospasm, may apply one or two drops of topical anesthetic).
- Determine if FB occurred from metal striking metal, as this may suggest possibility of an intraocular FB.
- Look for foreign objects by slit lamp examination.
- Evert upper and lower eyelids to identify additional FBs (if there is no evidence of perforation to the globe).
- Place fluorescein on corneal surface and examine for aqueous leakage through wound (possible Seidel's sign).
- Dilated retinal examination to rule out intraocular FB.
- CT scan or B-scan ultrasound of the eye and orbit if suggestive of an intraocular or intraorbital FB and not found on examination.

■ Treatment

- Place topical anesthetic (e.g., proparacaine, one to two drops) and irrigate if multiple superficial FBs present.
- Extract FB at the slit lamp using a fine-gauge needle (25G), cotton-tipped applicator, or jeweler's forceps.
- If a rust ring is present, remove with an ophthalmic drill and treat resulting corneal abrasion (see p. 36).
- After removing the FB, consider:

-Artificial tears, antibiotic ointment, or patching
-Topical NSAID (e.g., ketorolac tromethamine or diclofenac sodium, one drop four times per day) or oral acetaminophen for pain
-Short acting cycloplegic drugs (e.g., cyclopentolate 1%, one drop 1 to 4 times per day) for pain or photophobia

■ **Follow-up**

• Check after one week for conjunctival FB.
• For corneal FBs, check every 2 days until the epithelial defect is healed.
• Perform gonioscopy after healing to rule out anterior chamber angle damage.
• Advise patients to wear safety goggles when there is a risk of objects entering the eye, as in sports, operating drilling machinery, or construction work.

Chemical Burns

Chemical burns are caused by exposure of the eye/eyelid to any chemical substances. All chemical burns should be considered as a serious injury that may lead to irreversible damage to the eye tissues. The concentration of the exposed substance, the duration of its contact with the eye tissues, and the delay in time irrigation is initiated are all factors in determining the degree of damage.
    There are several types of toxic substances causing injury:

• Alkaline burns
  -Mostly caused by ammonia, lye, and lime
  -Most severe and serious chemical burn
  -Penetrate the epithelium, stroma, and endothelium
• Acid burns
  -Often result from exposure to car battery contents
  -Usually limited to the epithelial surface
• Irritants
  -Substances that have a neutral pH (e.g., household detergents)
  -Often cause discomfort rather than serious damage

■ **History**

• Recent history of irritant/chemical coming in contact with eye/lids
• Various degrees of pain
• Redness, tearing, and irritation
• Inability to keep the eye open
• Deterioration of vision
• Sensitivity to light (photophobia) and halos around lights

■ Clinical Manifestations

- Depending on the severity of the burn, the following signs are present in various degrees:
  - Excessive blood in the eye
  - Corneal epithelial defect
  - Edema of the bulbar conjunctiva associated with swelling around the cornea (chemosis)
  - Cells and flare in the AC on slit lamp examination
- Burns on periocular skin
- In very severe burns (e.g., alkali)
  - Corneal edema/opacification
  - Necrotic retinopathy from direct penetration of alkali through sclera
  - Increased IOP

■ Differential Diagnosis

- Corneal abrasion: usually there is an epithelial defect that stains with fluorescein on slit lamp examination; history helps differentiation.
- Herpes simplex keratitis: usually unilateral and sometimes associated with a vesicular skin rash and follicular conjunctivitis.
- Corneal ulcer (Plate 3): usually seen as a focal opacity/infiltrate in the corneal stroma on slit lamp examination.

■ Diagnostic Evaluation

- History is the key for diagnosis. History should focus on type of chemical, time of injury, duration of exposure to the substance, and duration of previous irrigation.
- Slit-lamp examination with fluorescein staining to look for epithelial defects.
- Check IOP (may be elevated in severe burns). May need to use a Tono-Pen in severe, damaged, or edematous corneas.
- Evert eyelids to rule out retained FBs.

■ Treatment

- Implement immediate treatment (flush), even before checking vision.
- Instant and copious fluid irrigation with saline of the affected eye for at least 30 minutes is the first step in management.
- Litmus paper should be used to test the eye's pH 5 minutes after completion of irrigation.
- Irrigation should be stopped when neutral pH is achieved. Reirrigate if pH is elevated.
- Removal of debris or any necrotic corneal or conjunctival tissue using a cotton-tipped applicator moistened with antibiotic solution. Evert eyelids and sweep fornices.

- Liberal use of artificial tears (e.g., Genteal, Systane, Refresh Tears, one drop 1 to 10 times per day).
- Use a strong cycloplegic agent (e.g., 0.25% scopolamine); avoid vasoconstrictors.
- Administer antibiotic ointment every 1 to 2 hours (e.g., erythromycin).
- Lower IOP if elevated.

  In more severe cases:

- A pressure patch should be considered. A topical corticosteroid during the first week following trauma may be administered, and an oral narcotic analgesic may be used as needed.

▓ Follow-up

- Monitor daily.
- Medications should be continued until the defect is healed.
- Monitoring of IOP is crucial because IOP spikes may occur as a late complication due to blockage of the trabecular meshwork by inflammatory debris.
- May need long-term liberal use of artificial tears/ointment.
- Discontinue any topical steroids within 7 to 10 days to avoid corneal melt.

Traumatic Iritis

Inflammation of the iris as a result of blunt trauma directed to the eye

▓ History

- Slow onset of a dull/throbbing pain after a recent history of ocular trauma
- Sensitivity to light (photophobia) and tearing
- May have blurred vision

▓ Clinical Manifestations

- White blood cells and flare in the AC (Plate 1)
- Pain when shining light into the affected or unaffected eye
- Often low IOP
- Conjunctival injection
- Smaller pupil in the affected eye (larger if iris sphincter tears present)
- Occasionally decreased vision

▓ Differential Diagnosis

- Traumatic corneal abrasion: associated with irregular lesions on the corneal epithelium with fluorescein dye. Usually no AC reaction.

- Traumatic retinal detachment: history of flashes of light after blunt trauma. Pigmented cells may be seen in the AC or anterior vitreous. Ophthalmoscopy reveals retinal detachment.
- Anterior uveitis (Plate 1): AC reaction but no history of trauma.
- Traumatic microhyphema: may see red blood cells (RBCs) in the AC.

▓ Diagnostic Evaluation
- Full eye examination with dilated fundus examination
- IOP evaluation and monitoring

▓ Treatment
- Cycloplegic agent (e.g., cyclopentolate 1%, one drop two to four times per day) is the key until the condition is resolved.
- Addition of steroid drops (e.g., prednisolone acetate 1%, one drop every 1 to 6 hours) may help pain, but do not use if there is a corneal defect.

▓ Follow-up
- Follow-up within a few days of trauma.
- Add steroid drops, if no improvement is achieved, within 1 week after the trauma occurred.
- Discontinue cycloplegic agent when symptoms resolve.
- 3 to 6 weeks after trauma:
  - Perform gonioscopy (see Figure 2-6) of the AC angle to rule out damage (e.g., angle recession).
  - Examine the retina (with scleral depression) to rule out retinal breaks or detachment.

Traumatic Hyphema

Hemorrhage in the AC caused by blunt trauma (e.g., assault, air bag injury) to the globe (Plate 4). Trauma stresses the AC angle, leading to damage and rupture of the iris and/or ciliary vessels. Angle recession, a separation between the longitudinal and circular muscle fibers of the ciliary muscle, may be an associated finding in this condition and may result in the development of glaucoma. The amount of blood in the AC varies from microscopic hemorrhage to total hyphema with no visible iris.

Blood in the AC may be classified as:

- Microhyphema: only see circulating RBCs
- Hyphema: blood is layered and/or clot is visible (Plate 4)

■ History
- History of blunt trauma
- Pain; blurred vision

■ Clinical Manifestations
- Reduced visual acuity
- Slit lamp examination reveals blood (RBCs) in AC

■ Risk Factors
- Systemic diseases such as sickle cell disease/trait, blood dyscrasia (leukemia, von Willebrand's disease), thrombotic disorder, pregnancy, renal disease
- Medications (i.e., warfarin, aspirin)

■ Differential Diagnosis
- Blunt rupture of the globe: may be associated with a variety of signs such as low IOP and shallow AC. History of a sharp object penetrating the globe is usually present.
- Intraocular tumor: CT scan is diagnostic. Symptoms vary according to the location and size of tumor. Papilledema may be present.
- Intraocular surgery: history of recent eye surgery and no history of trauma is present.
- Iris or corneal wound neovascularization: leaky and fragile new blood vessels are seen on the iris/cornea wound. No history of trauma is detected.
- Herpes simplex or zoster iritis: skin involvement is often present characterized by clear painful vesicles that follow a typical distribution on the body surface.

■ Diagnostic Evaluation
- Ascertain if there is a history of trauma.
- Perform a complete ophthalmic exam to rule out ruptured globe or other injuries. If able, perform dilated retinal examination; do not perform scleral depression as pressure on globe may cause a rebleed of the hyphema. Avoid gonioscopy initially for the same reason.
- Check visual acuity and IOP.
- Evaluate changes in corneal clarity. The presence of blood in the AC may result in corneal bloodstaining caused by infiltration of degraded erythrocytes, hemoglobin, and hemosiderin. The earliest sign of corneal bloodstaining is a yellowish discoloration of the deep corneal stroma.

- Measure the hyphema in terms of height or percentage of chamber filled with blood.
- Check for clotted as opposed to unclotted blood.
- Quantify free-floating RBCs (1+ to 4+).
- Check for a history of bleeding disorders, sickle cell hemoglobinopathy, or anticoagulant therapy (e.g., heparin, warfarin, or aspirin).

■ Treatment

The treatment for traumatic hyphema is controversial. Major goals for therapy are to prevent rebleeding and to control IOP.

- Bed rest with elevation of patient's head to 30 degrees to facilitate settling of hyphema. No strenuous activity.
- Topical steroids (e.g., prednisolone acetate 1%, one drop four times per day) for photophobia or to control inflammation.
- Cycloplegic drops (e.g., atropine 1% one to three times per day).
- Antifibrinolytic agents (i.e., aminocaproic acid 50 mg/kg PO q 4h for five days or tranexamic acid) are controversial in terms of their effectiveness in preventing rebleeds.
- Control IOP as needed: preferably with beta blockers (e.g., timolol 0.5% gel forming solution, one drop qd) or α-agonists (e.g., brimonidine 0.15%, one drop twice per day). Avoid carbonic anhydrase inhibitors (e.g., dorzolamide, brinzolamide) as they may increase the chance of rebleed because they decrease AC pH and increase sickling.
- Institute aggressive IOP reduction in sickle cell and sickle trait (IOP greater than 25 mm Hg) because these patients are at high risk for optic nerve damage.
- Avoid aspirin-containing drugs.
- Protect the eye with a shield to help blood settle.
- Sickle cell screening in black patients.
- Surgical intervention (e.g., paracentesis or AC washout) is needed if the IOP is elevated for a long time (more than 1 week), there is evidence of corneal staining, or there is a large clot or total blood in the AC.

■ Follow-up

- In uncomplicated simple cases, patients may be treated on an outpatient basis.
- All cases should be followed up on a daily basis.
- In complicated cases, patients should be hospitalized and treated as required.
- Perform dilated retinal examination to rule out retinal detachment and gonioscopy to rule out angle recession 1 month after trauma.

■ **Complications**

• Rebleeding
• Peripheral anterior synechiae, increased incidence with prolonged hyphema
• Elevated IOP, acutely due to:
  -Occlusion of trabecular meshwork by clot or inflammatory cells
  -Pupillary block
• Elevated IOP also increases risk of developing optic atrophy
• Corneal blood staining—more common in larger hyphemas
• Secondary glaucoma (e.g., angle recession glaucoma)

Blowout Fracture of the Orbit

Blowout fractures involve the orbital bones and are caused by blunt trauma to the orbit. The typical blowout fracture occurs when an object that has a circumference greater than the anterior orbital bones, such as a fist or baseball, strikes the orbital rim. The medial orbital wall and orbital floor are the most commonly affected sites, and injury there can result in entrapment of the medial rectus and inferior rectus muscles, respectively. Medial wall fractures often occur in association with floor fractures and rarely independently. In the setting of an orbital fracture one should always consider the possibility of ocular injuries such as damage to the sclera or cornea, lens dislocation, hyphema, vitreous hemorrhage, retinal detachment, or optic nerve injury.

■ **History**

• Pain at point of impact and potentially with eye movements (especially vertical eye movements).
• Binocular double vision (diplopia) because of entrapment of an extraocular muscle. Diplopia resolves when one eye is covered.
• Visual blurring and eyelid swelling.

■ **Clinical Manifestations**

• Extraocular motility restriction: upward and downward gaze can be simultaneously defective. If there is medial wall involvement, horizontal motility may be affected as well.
• Exophthalmos—protrusion of the globe—initially due to hemorrhage and edema.
• Globe ptosis (sinking of the globe inferiorly in the orbit).
• Enophthalmos—recession of the globe within the orbit—is more apparent days after the fracture with resolution of edema/hemorrhage.

- Periorbital edema, bruising, crepitus (crackling sound upon palpation of the lid due to air in the skin from the ethmoid sinus), tenderness.
- Hypoesthesia of the ipsilateral cheek and upper lip (distribution of infraorbital nerve—CN V_2).
- Nose bleeding.

Risk Factors
- Athletics: boxing, baseball, tennis, football
- Car accidents

Differential Diagnosis
- Orbital edema without a blowout fracture: usually resolves in a week. No fractures are detected on x-ray.
- Cranial nerve palsy: ocular movement restriction present, but CT scan or x-ray film reveals no fractures. Forced-duction testing reveals no restriction.

Diagnostic Evaluation
- Complete ophthalmic examination for signs of ocular injury including rupture, traumatic iritis, hyphema, or retinal/choroidal damage.
- Check movements of extraocular muscles. If restriction present for more than 7 to 10 days, perform forced-duction test to detect if muscle is entrapped.
- Measure for globe displacement with exophthalmometer.
- Check IOP.
- Perform CT scan (axial and coronals) of orbits if uncertain of diagnosis, or if suspect orbital roof fracture, or considering surgical repair.

Treatment
- Broad-spectrum oral antibiotics (e.g., erythromycin 250 mg PO four times per day or cephalexin 250 mg PO four times per day for 7 to 10 days).
- Consider oral steroids (e.g., prednisone 20–60 mg PO every day) for 7 to 10 days to decrease swelling and nasal decongestants for 1 to 2 weeks.
- Ice packs over affected area for 24 to 48 hours.
- Inform patient not to blow nose.
- Surgical intervention should be considered after 10 to 14 days if:
  - The patient exhibits diplopia for distance fixation and/or reading that does not improve within approximately 2 weeks
  - Large or complicated defects are present
  - The patient has unacceptable cosmetic issues relating to the fracture

Note: Surgical repair is usually not indicated the first 2 weeks because orbital edema may improve with resolution of diplopia/enophthalmos.

■ Follow-up

- Monitor for diplopia, enophthalmos, and the development of associated ocular injuries. If diplopia/enophthalmos persists after 2 weeks, entrapment of orbital contents or large displaced fracture may be present. Surgical repair may be considered at this point.
- Check the AC angle (gonioscopy) to rule out angle recession.
- Perform dilated retinal examination 1 month after trauma to rule out retinal detachment.

Traumatic Optic Neuropathy

Damage to the optic nerve may occur as a consequence of direct or indirect trauma. After an injury to the forehead, traumatic forces may be transmitted via the orbital bones to the optic canal. This may result in fracture of the optic canal or swelling of the blood vessels supplying the optic nerve within the canal.

■ History

- Acute, often persistent, loss of vision often accompanied by a recent history of trauma to the eye, periocular area, or forehead
- Occasionally, lucid interval followed by a drop in vision due to optic nerve swelling or hemorrhage
- Pain to the traumatized area

■ Clinical Manifestations

- Relative afferent pupillary defect (RAPD) in the affected eye not explained by ocular pathology.
- Poor color vision or visual field defect may be present in the affected eye.
- Usually normal appearance of optic disc initially.
- Optic disc cupping/pallor may develop in a few weeks (Plate 5).

■ Differential Diagnosis (of Causes of RAPD)

- Intracranial trauma: may involve the optic chiasm, in which case bilateral visual field defects may develop. CT scan helps differentiate.
- Compressive optic neuropathy: history of slowly progressive central loss of vision. RAPD is detected.

- Commotio retinae: disruption of retinal photoreceptors secondary to blunt trauma. It is associated with retinal edema and hemorrhage with a whitish gray central retinal lesion on ophthalmoscopic examination. Usually affects the posterior pole and resolves gradually.
- Vitreous hemorrhage: obscured view of the retina on dilated fundus examination and possible mild RAPD.
- Functional (nonphysiologic) loss of vision: normal ocular examination without RAPD.

■ Diagnostic Evaluation

- Full eye examination including pupillary examination to rule out RAPD. Must also rule out penetrating injury or ruptured globe.
- Visual field and color vision testing
- CT scan of the head/orbit to rule out fracture of optic canal or intraorbital FB.
- B-scan ultrasound for high suspicion of FBs not seen on CT scan.

■ Treatment

- High-dose intravenous steroids (e.g., methylprednisolone 250 mg IV every six hours for 12 doses) in the acute phase; then oral prednisone (60–80 mg PO every day).
- An oral antiulcer medication (e.g., ranitidine 150 mg PO twice per day) is often given concurrently with a steroid.
- Systemic antibiotics may be considered in orbit-penetrating injuries or fractures of the sinus wall (e.g., cefazolin 1 gm IV every eight hours).
- Surgery, if pathologic lesion found on CT and vision is decreasing:
  - Decompression surgery to the optic canal
  - Surgery to remove FBs from the orbit
  - Surgery to remove fragments compressing the optic nerve

■ Follow-up

- Monitor visual function including acuity, pupillary reaction, and color daily.
- If decreased vision after stopping/decreasing steroids, restart/increase steroids as before.
- Follow-up with perimetry a few months after the event.
- Refer patient to internist if placed on high-dose steroids.

5 Pediatric Ophthalmology

Thomas E. Bournias, MD

LEUKOCORIA (WHITE PUPILLARY REFLEX)

The normal pupillary reflex is reddish owing to light reflecting off the retina (which is red-orange) back through the pupil. If the pupil is obstructed or there is a lesion on the retina, a white reflex, termed leukocoria, may result (Plate 6).

■ Clinical Manifestations

- A child may be born or may develop a white reflex in one or both eyes.

■ Differential Diagnosis

- Retinoblastoma: most common intraocular tumor of childhood. Appears in the retina as a white nodular mass that may assume different forms, including extension into the vitreous, underlying a retinal detachment, or a diffusely spreading lesion masquerading as uveitis. May be unilateral, bilateral, or multilateral (involving the pineal gland). There is often a positive family history. Disease is usually diagnosed at 12 to 24 months of age. Strabismus is seen in one fourth of cases. Iris neovascularization may be present as well as pseudohypopyon (layered cells inferiorly in the anterior chamber). Vitreous seeding may also occur.
- Retinopathy of prematurity (ROP): A vascular abnormality of the retina usually resulting from low birth weight (less than 1500 g). ROP tends to occur in premature children who received supplemental oxygen. Retinal detachment results in leukocoria. It is usually bilateral.
- Coat's disease: A vascular abnormality of the retina resulting in multifocal areas of leakage of yellow intraretinal and subretinal exudates from outpouchings of the retinal vasculature. Leukocoria may appear from the resulting exudative retinal detachment. Primarily occurs in males in the first two decades of life, with more severity if it presents in the first decade.

Genetics is sporadic (no family history). Typically unilateral with only very rare bilateral cases.

- Congenital cataract: Unilateral or bilateral opacity of the lens present at birth. May be associated with a systemic disorder or a positive family history.

- Persistent hyperplastic primary vitreous (PHPV): A developmental abnormality with fibroglial and vascular proliferation in the vitreous cavity. The eye is usually smaller than normal. May be associated with cataract, glaucoma, and retinal detachment. There may be a fibrovascular membrane behind the lens that places traction on the ciliary processes. Family history is negative and it is almost always unilateral. It is present at birth but diagnosis can be delayed until later in childhood.

- Toxocariasis: A nematode infection in the posterior pole or peripheral retina often appearing as a localized, white, elevated granuloma. There are usually no signs of inflammation, but infection can appear as diffuse endophthalmitis with an inflamed globe. Vitreous traction bands associated with macular dragging and tractional retinal detachment may be seen. It is typically unilateral and primarily diagnosed between the ages of 3 and 10 years. A history of contact with dogs may be elicited.

- Retinal astrocytoma: A benign, flat to slightly elevated, yellow-white lesion on the retina that may be associated with calcification. It may be associated with tuberous scleroses and occasionally with giant drusen. It is rarely associated with neurofibromatosis.

- Others: retinal detachment, uveitis, myelinated nerve fiber layer.

■ Diagnostic Evaluation

- Determine the age of onset or if there is a family history or a history of contact with dogs (toxocariasis). Inquire if there is a history of prematurity or low birth weight with supplemental oxygen (ROP).

- Examination: Look for a small eye (seen in PHPV) by measuring the diameter of the cornea. On slit lamp examination look for evidence of neovascularization of the iris (retinoblastoma) or cataract (PHPV). Carefully inspect the retina and anterior vitreous on dilated fundus examination.

- Systemic examination with pediatrician in cases of congenital cataract, retinal astrocytoma, and retinoblastoma.

- B-scan ultrasound to differentiate PHPV, retinoblastoma, cataract.

- CT or MRI of the brain to detect evidence of retinoblastoma (pineal gland), especially in bilateral cases or when there is a positive family history.

- *Toxocara:* paracentesis of anterior chamber may demonstrate eosinophils **(caution: paracentesis in patient with retinoblastoma may lead to dissemination of tumor cells)**; serum enzyme-linked immunosorbent assay demonstrates positive titer in most infected patients.
- Examination under anesthesia (EUA) in uncooperative individuals, especially when considering diagnosis of retinoblastoma, ROP, toxocariasis, or Coat's disease.

■ Treatment

- Retinoblastoma: enucleation is the usual treatment for large tumors. Laser photocoagulation, cryotherapy, and irradiation may be implemented with smaller and more anterior tumors. Chemotherapy is employed in cases of metastasis. Survival decreases significantly if tumor is found in the optic nerve.
- ROP: managed with laser photocoagulation and/or cryotherapy if sufficient extraretinal fibrovascular proliferation is present in association with "plus disease" (a critical prognostic sign demonstrating engorged veins and tortuous arteries in the posterior pole). Retinal detachments are repaired if present. Recent studies have demonstrated better long-term vision with earlier treatment.
- Coat's disease: laser photocoagulation and/or cryotherapy to leaking vessels. Surgery to repair retinal detachment if necessary.
- Congenital cataract surgery is performed within days to weeks of diagnosis to hopefully prevent irreversible amblyopia. After cataract extraction, the child is treated for amblyopia (see p. 56) until the age of about 10 years. Any associated conditions, such as glaucoma, are managed and the child is referred to a pediatrician for management of any underlying systemic disorder.
- PHPV: cataract surgery and possible excision of vitreal membrane. Manage amblyopia if present.
- Toxocariasis: topical steroids to control mild or anterior segment inflammation. In cases of moderate to severe inflammation, consider periocular injection of depot steroid (e.g., triamcinolone 20–40 mg) during EUA. May consider systemic steroids (e.g., prednisone 10–40 mg PO every day). May perform surgical vitrectomy if condition does not improve or worsens with medical therapy or when vitreoretinal traction bands form.
- Retinal astrocytoma: observe.

■ Follow-up

- Varies, depending on the condition.
- Retinoblastoma patients should follow-up with an oncologist due to significant mortality rate.

- Children with amblyopia should be followed and treated closely (see p. 56).

STRABISMUS

Strabismus is a misalignment of the two eyes in which both eyes are not simultaneously directed toward an object. Both concomitant (nonparalytic) and incomitant (restrictive or paralytic) forms may be considered. Concomitant strabismus demonstrates approximately equal misalignment in all directions of gaze. The extraocular muscles (EOMs) function normally. This form of strabismus usually occurs in childhood. Strabismus amblyopia may result because of suppression to overcome double vision. Concomitant strabismus may occur in an adult with a blind eye (usually drifts outward in an adult, inward in a child) or from serious neurologic disease.

Incomitant strabismus demonstrates various degrees of misalignment in different directions of gaze. There is usually a malfunction of the EOMs or nerve, or a mechanical restriction of movement. This type of strabismus may result from cranial nerve paresis, restrictive ophthalmopathy (e.g., thyroid disease), or trauma (e.g., blowout fracture).

The most common deviations are esodeviations and exodeviations.

Esodeviations in Children

Inward turning of the eye. The corneal light reflex demonstrates a reflection on the temporal aspect of the cornea of the deviating eye.

▨ Clinical Manifestations
- Either eye turns inward (i.e., cross-eyed).
- During the cover-uncover test, the nonfixating eye turns outward to refixate straight ahead when the fixating eye is covered.
- Possible overaction of the inferior oblique muscles resulting in a vertical deviation.
- May develop amblyopia (usually in the nonfixating eye).
- Demonstrates both comitant and incomitant deviations:
  - Comitant esotropic deviations:
    - Congenital (infantile) esotropia: angle of esodeviation usually large (more than 40 prism diopters). Deviation is equal at distance and near fixation. Amblyopia usually develops in nonfixating eye (may not have amblyopia if alternating fixation). Refractive error typical for age (slightly hyperopic). Manifests by 6 months of age. Often a positive family history.

-Accommodative esotropia: convergent deviation of the eyes associated with stimulation of the accommodative reflex. Manifests on average at age 2.5 years.

-Sensory deprivation esotropia: an esodeviation in a patient with a condition or monocular or binocular lesion that precludes good vision (e.g., cataract, anisometropia, corneal opacity, retinal scar or tumor, etc.).

-Divergence insufficiency: convergent deviation that is greater at distance than near fixation. Diagnosis of exclusion. Must rule out divergence paralysis secondary to trauma or pontine tumor.

-Incomitant esodeviations: such as isolated sixth-nerve palsy, Duane's syndrome, hydrocephalus, etc.

■ Differential Diagnosis

- Pseudoesotropia: eyes appear esotropic, but no misalignment discovered during cover-uncover testing. Usually, prominent epicanthal folds, a wide nasal bridge, or a small interpupillary distance is present. Corneal light reflex is also normal.

- Duane's syndrome: motility disorder where there is limited abduction or adduction or both. On attempted adduction, the eyelid fissure narrows and the globe retracts.

- Isolated sixth-nerve palsy: affected eye does not turn outward (temporally), but no restriction is found on forced-duction testing. Etiologic factors include benign postviral condition, pontine glioma, and trauma.

- Brown's syndrome: motility disorder where the adducted eye has limitation of elevation. Usually, the eyes are straight in primary gaze and elevation is normal in abduction. Ten percent of cases are bilateral. May be congenital or acquired. Acquired cases are usually secondary to trauma, surgery, or inflammation (especially around the trochlea).

- Nystagmus blockage syndrome: esotropia associated with nystagmus. Nystagmus is exacerbated when the fixating eye is abducted and lessened in adduction. When one eye is occluded, the head turns toward the uncovered eye (in order to lessen the nystagmus).

- Möbius' syndrome: unilateral or bilateral esotropia, with inability to abduct the involved eye. Facial nerve or other cranial nerve palsies may be present.

■ Diagnostic Evaluation

- Determine when the eyes were first noted to be crossed. Ascertain if the deviation is constant or intermittent or straightened by glasses. Examine old photographs and determine if there was a history of trauma.

- Determine if amblyopia is present by checking visual acuity of each eye individually with refraction and pinhole.
- Perform ocular motility examination to detect restricted movements.
- Determine refractive error with manifest and cycloplegic retinoscopy.
- Check for a relative afferent pupillary defect (RAPD).
- Perform complete ocular examination to determine if sensory deprivation is present.
- Neurologic consultation and head CT/MRI to rule out intracranial lesion if divergence insufficiency or paralysis is present.
- If esodeviation is incomitant and abduction is limited, then consider a diagnosis of one of the syndromes in the differential diagnosis above (except pseudoesotropia).

■ Treatment

- Correct hyperopia of greater than +2.00 diopters in all cases.
- Manage amblyopia (if present) by patching the better-seeing eye (see treatment of Amblyopia, pp. 57–58).
- Congenital esotropia: Perform corrective muscle surgery when vision is equal in both eyes or to preserve stereo vision.
- Accommodative esotropia: Correct the hyperopia. Consider bifocals if the child has straight distance vision but esotropia at near (high AC/A ratio) with full correction. Glasses should be worn full time.
- Sensory deprivation esotropia: Give full cycloplegic correction and use protective glasses (e.g., polycarbonate) if poor vision exists in one eye. Address the cause of poor vision. Muscle surgery is cosmetic only.

■ Follow-up

- Measure the degree of deviation with prisms (with glasses on) at each visit.
- Evaluate and manage amblyopia at each visit.
- In cases without amblyopia, evaluate in 1 to 6 months if there is no change in glasses prescription. Reevaluate in 3 to 6 weeks if a new prescription was given.
- If residual esotropia is present with glasses, attempt to add more plus power without blurring the patient's vision.
- May have to decrease plus power after 5 to 7 years of age as hyperopia usually decreases at this time.

Exodeviations in Children

Outward turning of the eye. The corneal light reflex demonstrates a reflection on the nasal aspect of the cornea of the deviating eye.

▣ Clinical Manifestations

- Either eye turns outward, constantly or intermittently.
- During the cover-uncover test, the uncovered eye turns inward when the fixating eye is covered.
- May demonstrate a vertical deviation (with overaction of the superior or inferior oblique muscles).
- May develop amblyopia.
- There are many types of exodeviations:
  - Intermittent exotropia: onset is from infancy to 4 years. Tends to be progressive in frequency, but amblyopia is rare. Most common type of exodeviation in children.
  - Third-nerve palsy: exotropia with limitation of eye movements superiorly, medially, and inferiorly. Usually associated with ptosis of the exotropic eye.
  - Sensory deprivation exotropia: a poor seeing eye that turns out over time.
  - Myasthenia gravis: limitation of eye movement and ptosis may vary at different times of day. Edrophonium chloride (e.g., Tensilon) test result may be positive.
  - Duane's syndrome (type 2): limited adduction only
  - Convergence insufficiency: exodeviation at near fixation, but no deviation at distance fixation. Patients often complain of headaches and blurred vision while reading. Symptoms usually develop after 10 years of age.

▣ Differential Diagnosis

- Pseudoexotropia: patient appears to have an exodeviation, but cover-uncover testing reveals no deviation. There is also a normal corneal light reflex. Causes include:
  - Wide interpupillary distance
  - Temporal dragging of the macula (e.g., toxocariasis, ROP)

▣ Diagnostic Evaluation

- Determine if amblyopia is present by checking best corrected vision in each eye with refraction (manifest and cycloplegic).
- Check ocular motility to determine if Duane's syndrome or restricted eye movements are present.
- Check for RAPD.
- Determine if proptosis is present with Hertel exophthalmometer.
- Measure the amount of exodeviation with prisms straight ahead (primary position) and in all positions of gaze at both near and distance fixation.
- Consider edrophonium chloride (e.g., Tensilon) test if myasthenia gravis suspected.

▦ Treatment
- Correct significant refractive error.
- Manage amblyopia if present (see treatment of amblyopia, p. 57).
- Muscle surgery to maintain binuclear fusion or to correct any significant abnormal head position in primary gaze.

▦ Follow-up
- If amblyopia is present, follow up as described below for treatment of amblyopia.
- Every 4 to 6 months if no amblyopia is present; sooner if deviation worsens or increases in frequency.

AMBLYOPIA

A unilateral (or, rarely, bilateral) decrease in visual acuity (with best spectacle correction) that is not a direct result of any structural abnormality of the eye or posterior visual pathway. It occurs in about 2% to 4% of the population in North America. Amblyopia results from abnormal visual development before the age of 10 years. There are three main causes.

▦ Etiology
- Anisometropia: a large difference in refractive error (usually greater than three diopters) between the two eyes.
- Strabismus: the eyes are not straight, with the deviating eye (nonfixating eye) demonstrating worse vision.
- Form deprivation or occlusion: anything that diminished the quality of images transmitted to the brain. May result from ptosis (drooping lid) or media opacity secondary to a corneal scar, cataract, PHPV, etc. Some cases may be iatrogenic (from patching therapy over the normal eye of an amblyopic patient).

▦ History
- Decreased vision (primarily one eye)
- A history of patching, strabismus, or muscle surgery as a child

▦ Clinical Manifestations
- Worse vision in one eye not corrected with refraction or explained by an organic cause.
- Develops during first 10 years of life without subsequent deterioration.
- During examination of visual acuity, individual letters may be read better than the entire line (crowding phenomenon).

- Significant RAPD is very rare, even when amblyopia is significant.

■ Diagnostic Evaluation
- Ascertain if there is a history of eye problems (e.g., misalignment), patching, or muscle surgery.
- Check vision and perform cycloplegic refraction to rule out anisometropia.
- Perform cover-uncover test to evaluate eye alignment and rule out strabismus.
- Perform complete eye examination to rule out organic cause of reduced vision.
- Examine pupils to determine if RAPD is present.

■ Treatment/Follow-up
- Eliminate if possible any obstacle to vision (e.g., cataract).
- Correct any significant refractive error.
- Force use of the poorer eye by limiting use of the better eye (in unilateral/asymmetric cases) via patching.
  - Children younger than 10 years:
    - Spectacle correction for significant anisometropia
    - Full-time patching over the better-seeing eye for 1 week per year of age (e.g., 2 weeks for a 2-year-old); then repeat the examination.
    - Patching, as above, is continued until the vision is equal in the two eyes or if vision is not improved after three rounds of patching (assuming compliance). Part-time patching (3 to 6 hr/day) may be considered until the age of 10 years if there is a recurrence.
    - Consider atropine ointment 0.5–1% three times per day in the better eye if there is noncompliance with patching. Patching is preferred and more effective, however.
    - If decreased vision in the patched eye results (occlusion amblyopia), patch the better-seeing eye for a short time (e.g., 1 day per year of age). Then repeat the examination.
    - If strabismus is present, consider strabismus surgery if there is poor stereo vision or when the vision is equal in both eyes.
  - Children older than 10 years:
    - Treatment is without benefit.
    - Wear protective glasses (e.g., polycarbonate lenses) if only one eye has good vision.

  Note: Amblyopia may occasionally occur bilaterally in cases of bilateral visual deprivation (e.g., high refractive errors or congenital cataracts).

- Pirate patches and patches worn over glasses are rarely as effective as patches that adhere to the skin and are directly worn over the eye.
- A large recent study demonstrated that with compliant full-time therapy, 97% of children may attain 20/40 visual acuity or better.

6

Neuro-Ophthalmology

Thomas E. Bournias, MD

Pupil

The pupil is the central portion of the iris plane. It both constricts (miosis) and dilates (mydriasis). Mydriasis is controlled by the dilator muscle, which is controlled primarily by sympathetic innervation. Miosis is controlled by the sphincter muscle, which primarily receives parasympathetic innervation.

■ Sympathetic Innervation

Sympathetic innervation (Figure 6-1) traverses a long path from the brain to the dilator muscle via the first-, second-, and third-order sympathetic innervation. The first-order neuron of the sympathetic chain begins in the ipsilateral posterolateral hypothalamus and traverses through the brain stem to synapse in the intermediolateral gray matter of the spinal cord at the level of C8, T1, and T2 (ciliospinal center of budge). The second-order neuron then exits the spinal cord and travels under the subclavian artery before passing over the pulmonary apex. It then passes through the stellate ganglion, without synapsing, to synapse in the superior cervical ganglion. Then, originating from the superior cervical ganglion, the third-order postganglionic neuron joins the internal carotid plexus, enters the cavernous sinus, and travels with the ophthalmic division of cranial nerve V (CN V) through the superior orbital fissure to the orbit and then to the dilator muscle.

■ Parasympathetic Innervation (Figure 6-2)

The sphincter muscle is composed of a circular band of smooth muscle fibers located near the pupillary margin. It has dual innervation, but it receives its primary innervation from parasympathetic fibers that originate in the nucleus of CN III. The sympathetic innervation to the sphincter muscle appears to serve an inhibitory role dilating the pupil in darkness. The parasympathetic pathway regulates the pupil size in different levels of lighting conditions.

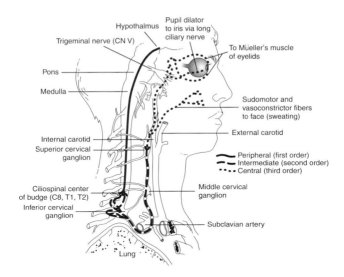

Figure 6-1 • The pathway of the first-, second-, and third-order neurons of the oculosympathetic pathway from the hypothalamus to the iris dilator muscle. Note the proximity of the apex of the lung to the sympathetic chain. Therefore, a Pancoast tumor may result in an ipsilateral Horner's syndrome.

Afferent Limb

The pupillary response to light originates in the rods and cones. The afferent pupillomotor fibers are transmitted via the optic nerve and hemidecussate at the chiasm. These fibers follow the visual sensory pathway through the optic tracts, exiting just before the lateral geniculate body (where the visual fibers synapse) to enter the brain stem by way of the brachium of the superior colliculus. The pupillomotor fibers synapse at the pretectal nuclei. The pretectal nuclei then project to both ipsilateral and contralateral Edinger-Westphal nuclei in the oculomotor nuclear complex in the midbrain.

Efferent Limb

The efferent pupillary fibers exit the Edinger-Westphal nucleus to join the third cranial nerve. Initially these fibers are located on the superior surface of the nerve. The third nerve rests on the edge of the tentorium cerebrum on its way to the cavernous sinus, where the uncal portion of the undersurface of the temporal lobe rests. Here, a supratentorial space-occupying mass may compress the efferent fibers (uncal herniation) and result in a dilated and fixed pupil (Hutchinson's pupil). The third nerve also travels lateral to the posterior communicating artery here and is

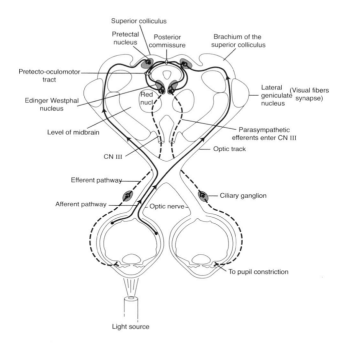

Figure 6-2 • The afferent and efferent parasympathetic pathway of the pupillary reaction to light. —— afferent; - - - - - efferent

also vulnerable to compression by an aneurysm, especially at the junction of the posterior communicating and the internal carotid arteries.

As the third nerve courses forward in the subarachnoid space and cavernous sinus, the pupillary fibers move down around the outside of the nerve to enter the inferior division of CN III. These efferent fibers then leave the inferior division of the third nerve and synapse at the ciliary ganglion. Parasympathetic postganglionic fibers are then distributed to the iris sphincter and ciliary body by way of the short ciliary nerves. Thus, light information presented to one eye is transmitted to both pupils equally.

An intact parasympathetic pathway results in a normal swinging flashlight test. The examiner projects light on the (for example) right eye and observes both pupils constrict. At this point, the examiner quickly swings the light to the left eye, which will remain constricted (except for some subsequent escape to an intermediate size). Consider an afferent pupillary defect (for example) in the left eye. After shining the light in the right eye resulting in constriction of both pupils, the light is swung over quickly to the opposite side, and the previously constricted left pupil will show anywhere from initial constriction with greater escape to immediate dilation (RAPD or Marcus Gunn pupil).

Anisocoria

During distance fixation and with constant, moderate, ambient illumination the pupils tend to be of equal and constant size. There is a small bilateral, symmetric, nonrhythmic variation in size (usually less than 1 mm) termed hippus. When shifting to near fixation, equal miosis of the pupils is noted. Miosis is also noted when bright light is placed before one or both eyes during distance fixation. This "light" miosis is equal to or greater than "near" miosis. About 20% of the population has clearly discernible pupils of unequal size (termed anisocoria).

■ Etiology

- Abnormal pupil is constricted:
  - Unilateral use of miotic eye drops such as pilocarpine
  - Iritis: anterior chamber cell and flare (Plate 1) usually present; may have eye pain or redness
  - Horner's syndrome: mild ipsilateral ptosis usually present with a positive cocaine test
  - Argyll Robertson pupil: secondary to syphilis, typically bilateral but usually with a mild degree of anisocoria
  - Long-standing Adie's tonic pupil: initially pupil is dilated in Adie's, but may constrict over time. It reacts poorly to light but occasionally mildly to prolonged near effort (convergence).
- Abnormal pupil is dilated:
  - Trauma to iris sphincter: may see transillumination defects at pupillary border on slit lamp examination.
  - Adie's tonic pupil: pupil is dilated in initial Adie's.
  - Unilateral use of mydriatic drop such as atropine: will not constrict to pilocarpine during first week.
  - Third-nerve palsy: associated with extraocular muscle palsies and ipsilateral ptosis. Pupil will react to regular strength pilocarpine (1%), but not to weaker strengths.
- Physiologic anisocoria: size difference between the two pupils is usually 1 mm or less. The pupils react normally to light, and anisocoria is the same in both light and dark situations.

■ Diagnostic Evaluation (Table 6-1)

- Ask when anisocoria was first noted and if associated with signs or symptoms or decreased vision. Examine old photographs.

■ TABLE 6-1 Pharmacologic Testing for Anisocoria

Condition	Pupil Pathology	Drug	Normal Pupil	Pathologic Pupil
Horner's syndrome	Constricted	Cocaine 4%–10%	Dilates	Fails to dilate
- Preganglionic	Constricted	Paredrine 1%	Dilates	Dilates
- Postganglionic	Constricted	Paredrine 1%	Dilates	Fails to dilate
Argyll Robertson pupil	Constricted	N/A	—	—
Adie's pupil	Dilated	Pilocarpine 0.05%–0.1%	No reaction	Constricts
CN III palsy	Dilated	Pilocarpine 1%	Constricts	Constricts
Pharmacologic pupil (e.g., atropine)	Dilated	Pilocarpine 1%	Constricts	Fails to constrict

Ascertain if there has been a history of eye drops or ointment use, ocular trauma, or syphilis.

- Ocular examination: Observe the pupillary size and try to determine which is the abnormal pupil. Pupils are normally 4 to 5 mm in younger people (slightly smaller in older individuals). Compare pupil sizes in light and dark if it is not obvious which is the abnormal pupil. If anisocoria is greater in dark, the smaller pupil is abnormal. The larger pupil is abnormal if anisocoria is greater in light. Determine the pupillary reaction to light and, if abnormal, test for convergence. Some conditions, such as dorsal midbrain syndrome (Parinaud's syndrome), Adie's or Argyll Robertson pupil, are associated with light—near dissociation (where the near reflex is intact with an abnormal light reflex). There is no condition in which the light reflex is normal but the near (convergence) reflex is abnormal. Examine the lids for ptosis and ocular motility for evidence of paralysis. Perform a slit lamp examination and evaluate the pupillary margin (to rule out trauma) and anterior chamber (to rule out iritis).
- If the abnormal pupil is small and there is an unequivocal increase in anisocoria in dim illumination with associated ptosis, Horner's syndrome is diagnosed. If the diagnosis is not obvious, Horner's syndrome may be confirmed by a cocaine test (see Horner's Syndrome on next page).
- If the abnormal pupil is large and there is no evidence of a third-nerve palsy (extraocular motility restriction associated with ptosis), then both pupils are tested with one to two drops of diluted pilocarpine 0.125% (prepared by diluting one part of pilocarpine 1% with seven parts saline solution). An Adie's

pupil constricts significantly more than the normal pupil after 15 minutes (see Adie's Tonic Pupil on p. 67). In a chronic Adie's pupil, the pupil may not react to dilute pilocarpine 0.125%.

- If pharmacologic dilation is suspected (e.g., atropine) or the pupil did not respond to pilocarpine 0.125%, one drop of pilocarpine 1% may be placed in both eyes. A pharmacologically dilated pupil will constrict much less and more slowly than a normal pupil.

■ Treatment/Follow-up

- For further information on managing the above causes of anisocoria, see Horner's Syndrome, Argyll Robertson Pupil, Adie's Tonic Pupil, and Isolated Third-Nerve Palsy on p. 68.

Horner's Syndrome

A defect of the sympathetic pathway resulting in ipsilateral miosis, ptosis, enophthalmos (apparent recession of the globe into the orbit), and possibly anhydrosis (lack of sweating).

■ Etiology

- First-order neuron: stroke (vertebrobasilar artery insufficiency); tumor.
- Second-order neuron: tumor (e.g., lung tumor, metastasis, thyroid adenoma, neurofibroma). Suspect Pancoast's tumor if arm pain present. In children, suspect neuroblastoma, lymphoma, or metastasis.
- Third-order neuron: headache (Raeder's paratrigeminal neuralgia, migraine, cluster), internal carotid dissection (superior cervical ganglion lies near the bifurcation of the carotid artery), herpes zoster virus, Tolosa-Hunt syndrome, otitis media.
- Congenital: trauma (e.g., Erb's palsy from delivery).

■ History

- Pupil size disparity (smaller pupil is abnormal), ipsilateral droopy eyelid (ptosis)
- Often asymptomatic

■ Clinical Manifestations

- Anisocoria (greater in dim illumination because smaller pupil unable to dilate well due to defective sympathetic innervation)
- Ipsilateral drooping of upper eyelid (ptosis) and elevated lower eyelid (reverse ptosis)

- Ipsilateral anhydrosis (loss of sweating ability)
- Iris heterochromia (lighter iris color in affected eye) in congenital cases
- Increased accommodation in involved eye
- Intact light and near reaction

■ Differential Diagnosis
- See Anisocoria above.

■ Diagnostic Evaluation
- Determine the duration of Horner's syndrome (old photographs may help). New-onset Horner's syndrome requires more extensive workup (an old Horner's syndrome is more likely to be benign). Ask about headache, arm pain, or previous stroke. Determine if there was a history of damage to the sympathetic chain such as previous surgery including thoracic, cardiac, thyroid, or neck or any head or neck trauma. Determine if there is a history of stroke, arm pain, or headache.
- Physical examination: Check for palpable supraclavicular nodes, thyroid enlargement, or a neck mass.
- Cocaine test if diagnosis is uncertain: place one drop of cocaine 4% to 10% in both eyes and repeat in 1 minute. After 15 minutes check pupillary size; if no change is present, place an additional drop in both eyes and reevaluate in another 15 minutes. A Horner's pupil will dilate less than the normal pupil (cocaine blocks reuptake of norepinephrine).
- Paredrine test (hydroxyamphetamine 1%): may be used when Horner's syndrome is confirmed to distinguish a first- and second-order (preganglionic) neuron disorder from a third-order (postganglionic) neuron disorder. Wait at least 24 hours if cocaine test was performed. Place one drop of hydroxyamphetamine 1% into both eyes, and repeat 1 minute later. If the Horner's pupil does not dilate to an equivalent amount as the normal eye, a third-order neuron lesion is present. (Paredrine releases norepinephrine from the presynaptic terminal.)
- Some of the following tests may be performed if a new-onset Horner's is discovered, a tumor is suspected, or a preganglionic lesion is present.
  - Chest x-ray or CT of lung with special attention to the apex
  - CT (axial and coronal) or MRI of brain and neck
  - CBC with differential
  - Lymph node biopsy in presence of lymphadenopathy
  - Carotid angiogram, magnetic resonance angiography (MRA), or carotid Doppler ultrasound in cases of neck pain where carotid dissection is suspected

■ Treatment
- Management of underlying disorder if possible
- Ptosis surgery if necessary

■ Follow-up
- As soon as possible in acute situation to rule out a life-threatening cause
- As soon as possible in a child with ptosis to treat for possible amblyopia (see amblyopia treatment, p. 57)
- Chronic Horner's syndrome is evaluated routinely.

Argyll Robertson Pupil

A rare syndrome that occurs in some patients with tertiary syphilis involving the central nervous system (CNS). Over time both pupils become small (less than 2 mm) and irregular. This is one of the rare situations where a very miotic pupil may react briskly.

■ Etiology
- Tertiary syphilis [positive fluorescent treponemal antibody, absorbed (FTA-ABS)]

■ History
- Usually asymptomatic

■ Clinical Manifestations
- Small, irregular pupils that react poorly to light but normally to convergence (light-near dissociation). Pupils dilate poorly.
- Initially unilateral, but later becomes bilateral. Often asymmetric.
- Normal vision.

■ Differential Diagnosis
- See Anisocoria above.

■ Diagnostic Evaluation
- Test pupillary reaction to light and convergence (determine if light-near dissociation exists).
- Look for evidence of interstitial keratitis on slit lamp examination.
- Look for uveitis, chorioretinitis, and papillitis on dilated fundus examination.
- Check FTA-ABS and rapid plasma reagin (RPR) or Venereal Disease Research Laboratory (VDRL) results.
- Possible lumbar puncture if positive diagnosis of syphilis.

■ **Treatment**
- See Chapter 11, Acquired Syphilis, p. 157
- The decision to treat is based on the presence of active disease and if the patient had previously been treated appropriately.

■ **Follow-up**
- Not emergent.
- Workup patient in a few days to 2 weeks to determine if syphilitic activity is present.

Adie's Tonic Pupil

Dilated pupil that appears to be benign in nature. The pupil may get smaller with time. The cause is unknown, but the ciliary ganglion has been found to have a dramatic reduction in ganglion cells.

■ **Etiology**
- Idiopathic
- Orbital trauma
- Infection with herpes zoster, varicella, syphilis
- May be bilateral in diabetes, chronic alcoholism, familial dysautonomia (Riley-Day syndrome)

■ **Epidemiology**
- 70% women
- 80% unilateral, second pupil may become involved later.

■ **History**
- Anisocoria, larger pupil dilated
- Blurred vision
- May be asymptomatic

■ **Clinical Manifestations**
- Irregularly dilated pupil.
- Affected pupil demonstrates minimal to no reaction to light and slow constriction to convergence with slow redilation afterwards (light-near dissociation).
- Affected pupil is supersensitive (constricts) to weak cholinergics (e.g., one drop of pilocarpine 0.125%).
- Normal dilation with mydriatics.
- Chronically, the involved pupil may become smaller than the normal pupil.
- Adie's syndrome: when associated with absent deep tendon reflexes (ankles and knees).

■ **Differential Diagnosis**

See Anisocoria above.

■ **Diagnostic Evaluation**

- See diagnostic evaluation for anisocoria for general workup.
- Examine the suspicious pupil with bright light at the slit lamp to confirm a pupil that reacts slowly and irregularly.
- Measure the size of each pupil as the patient fixates at distance. Check for a supersensitive pupil by placing one drop of pilocarpine 0.125% in both eyes.
- An Adie's tonic pupil constricts significantly more than the normal contralateral pupil. Occasionally, the supersensitivity may not be present immediately after developing an Adie's pupil; therefore, supersensitivity testing may be repeated 2 to 3 weeks later.
- Dilute pilocarpine may yield a positive result in Argyll Robertson pupil and familial dysautonomia.

Note: Parinaud's syndrome: may cause bilateral middilated pupils that react poorly to light but constrict normally during convergence (unlike Adie's), upgaze paralysis, convergence-retraction nystagmus, and lid retraction (Collier's sign). With these signs, perform an MRI to rule out pinealoma or other midbrain abnormality.

■ **Treatment**

- May treat with pilocarpine 0.125% two to four times per day to constrict the pupil for cosmetic purposes or to improve accommodation.

■ **Follow-up**

- Routine follow-up if diagnosis is certain
- If the patient is younger than 1 year, and Adie's pupil or supersensitivity is present, refer the patient to a pediatric neurologist to rule out familial dysautonomia.

Isolated Third-Nerve Palsy

Defect in CN III resulting in motility impairment (external ophthalmoplegia) and possibly impairment of pupillary reaction (internal ophthalmoplegia). Pupillary involvement may occur secondary to aneurysm, tumor, ischemia, trauma, or giant cell arteritis (GCA). The pupil is controlled by the efferent parasympathetics (miosis) that run in the inferior division of CN III, which innervates the medial and inferior recti.

■ History

- Double vision that disappears when one eye is occluded
- Ptosis (droopy eye lid) with/without pain

■ Clinical Manifestations

- Limitation of ocular movements, especially superior, inferior, and nasal.
- Ptosis may be present.
- Pupil may be dilated with diminished reactivity to light.
- Eye may appear to be looking down and/or out.
- May see aberrant regeneration (elevation of the upper lid and possibly constriction of the pupil with superior, medial, or inferior gaze). If this sign occurs spontaneously (primary), it may indicate a cavernous sinus aneurysm or tumor.

■ Differential Diagnosis

- GCA: pupil may or may not be involved but may develop ocular motility dysfunction.
- Myasthenia gravis: no pupil involvement; fluctuation in ptosis and diplopia; ptosis worsens with sustained gaze; positive result on edrophonium chloride (e.g., Tensilon) test.
- Thyroid eye disease: have lid retraction and not ptosis; may have ocular motility disorders. May have proptosis. Also may have injection over recti muscle insertions and resistance on forced-duction testing.
- Orbital inflammatory pseudotumor: idiopathic orbital inflammation with pain on eye movement. Patients may have double vision with restriction of ocular motility. May have proptosis and/or decreased vision.
- Internuclear ophthalmoplegia: unilateral or bilateral adduction deficit with horizontal nystagmus in the opposite abducting eye. A lesion of the medial longitudinal fasciculus. Ptosis is not present. Seen in multiple sclerosis.
- Chronic progressive ophthalmoplegia: pupil is spared. Patients demonstrate progressive bilateral ptosis and ocular motility deficits. May or may not have diplopia.
- Parinaud's syndrome: dorsal midbrain lesion with bilateral inability to look up and pupils demonstrating normal reaction to accommodation but abnormal reaction to light (light-near dissociation). There is no ptosis, and lid retraction and convergence-retraction nystagmus may be present.

■ Diagnostic Evaluation

- Ascertain if there is a history of trauma or medical illness such as diabetes, hypertension, or cancer.

- Complete ocular examination with careful attention to pupil examination. Check for ptosis and signs of aberrant regeneration.
- Check exophthalmometer for presence of proptosis.
- Check for signs of other cranial nerve abnormalities.
- Order immediate brain CT scan or MRI to rule out a mass/aneurysm if:
  - There is pupillary involvement.
  - The pupil is not involved but:
    - Other cranial nerves are involved.
    - The patient is younger than 50 years without a history of diabetes or hypertension.
    - The third-nerve palsy has been present for more than 3 months without improvement.
  - There is spontaneous aberrant regeneration.
- Check fasting blood sugar/Hb A_{1c} and blood pressure if suspicious of ischemic disease.
- Check ESR if suspicious of GCA.
- Check edrophonium chloride (e.g., Tensilon) test if suspicious of myasthenia gravis (and pupil is not involved).

■ Treatment
- Manage underlying abnormality or vascular disease if present.
- If double vision is present, may patch involved eye (patching not generally done in children under 10 years of age for fear of amblyopia).

■ Follow-up
- Pupil-involved third-nerve palsy: workup as described above and immediate hospitalization.
- Pupil-spared third-nerve palsy: workup as described and, if new, observe for 1 week. Recheck every 6 weeks.
- Normal function should return in about 3 months.
- If function is not restored by 3 months or additional neurologic abnormality results, an MRI of the brain is indicated.

Papilledema

Bilateral optic disc swelling caused by increased intracranial pressure

■ Etiology
- Intracranial tumors (primary and metastatic)
- Pseudotumor cerebri (benign intracranial hypertension): usually occurs in women, often overweight. CT scan or MRI of the brain is normal, but may have exotropia secondary to CN VI palsy.

- Aqueductal stenosis: may produce hydrocephalus
- Subdural and epidural hematoma: from trauma, especially if on anticoagulation therapy
- Subarachnoid hemorrhage: causes severe headache. May develop preretinal and vitreous hemorrhage (Terson's syndrome)
- Brain abscess: especially if HIV positive; may cause fever
- Arteriovenous malformation (AVM)

■ History

- Transient loss of vision (lasting seconds) usually bilateral and caused by changes in posture
- Decrease in visual acuity acutely (if associated with macular edema)
- Severe decrease of visual acuity and visual field defects with chronic papilledema (secondary to optic nerve pallor)
- Double vision (if CN VI palsy present)
- Headache, nausea, vomiting

■ Clinical Manifestations

- Early: bilateral, swollen, hyperemic optic nerves with blurring of the disc margin (Plate 7)
  - Normal pupil response to light and normal color vision.
  - Papillary and peripapillary retinal hemorrhages (often flame shaped) and cotton-wool spots may be present.
  - Dilated, tortuous retinal veins.
  - Absent venous pulsation at optic disc (absent in 20% of normal persons).
  - Visual field testing may reveal an enlarged blind spot.
- Chronic: optic atrophy (Plate 5)
  - Decreased central visual acuity and color vision
  - Esotropia (secondary to unilateral or bilateral sixth-nerve palsy)
  - Collateral vessels on the optic disk
  - Resolution of peripapillary hemorrhages and cotton-wool spots
  - Narrowing of peripapillary retinal vessels with peripapillary gliosis
  - Visual field defects

■ Differential Diagnosis (causes of bilateral disc edema)

- Pseudopapilledema: e.g., optic nerve drusen. Disc margins are sharp and vessels are not obscured. The neuroretinal rim is not hyperemic and the surrounding nerve fiber layer is normal.
- Malignant hypertensive retinopathy (Plate 8): fundus examination reveals bilateral narrowed arterioles with arteriovenous

nicking. There are associated scattered hemorrhages with cotton-wool spots. Blood pressure is extremely high.

- Ischemic optic neuropathy (ION): sudden, severe, unilateral loss in vision that may soon involve the second eye (e.g., GCA and nonarteritic ION). Optic nerve swelling is pale and not hyperemic.
- Diabetic papillitis: usually bilateral disc edema possibly associated with diabetic retinopathy changes. Typically seen in young persons with type I diabetes.
- Infiltration of the optic nerve: usually unilateral but can be bilateral. Seen in sarcoidosis, leukemia, tuberculosis, metastasis, and other inflammatory diseases. If seen in a leukemia patient, immediate radiation therapy is indicated to preserve vision.
- Graves' ophthalmopathy: other signs of thyroid dysfunction would be evident (see Chapter 11, Thyroid disease, p. 150).
- Leber's optic neuropathy: begins unilaterally but rapidly becomes bilateral. There is a rapid, progressive loss of vision with disc swelling associated with peripapillary telangiectasia that later becomes atrophic. Occurs primarily in men in their second to third decade of life. Family history may or may not be present.

■ Diagnostic Evaluation

- Determine if there is a history of systemic disease, especially hypertension, thyroid disease, and diabetes.
- Ophthalmic examination should include pupillary and color vision testing. Dilated fundus examination should carefully observe the vitreous for signs of inflammation, and the optic nerve appearance should be carefully noted.
- Check blood pressure.
- Immediate CT (axial and coronal) or MRI of the brain (and possibly the orbit) in all cases of bilateral disc edema (papilledema) to rule out a space occupying lesion.
- Lumbar puncture if CT/MRI result is unremarkable.

■ Treatment

- Address underlying cause.

■ Follow-up

- Initially weekly; later less frequently.
- Follow visual acuity and visual field carefully.

Optic Neuritis

An inflammation of the optic nerve of unknown cause associated with rapid deterioration of vision followed by a steady recovery.

■ **Etiology**

- Idiopathic
- Multiple sclerosis
- Viral infections, such as mononucleosis, herpes zoster, encephalitis, measles, mumps, chickenpox
- Granulomatous inflammations, such as syphilis, sarcoidosis, and tuberculosis
- Intraocular inflammations

■ **Epidemiology**

- Usually occurs between ages 20 to 45 years
- Occurs in nearly 100% of patients with long-standing multiple sclerosis

■ **History**

- Visual loss usually deteriorating over days until about 1 week (visual loss may deteriorate rarely over hours and may be subtle to extreme).
- Usually unilateral, 90% with orbital pain especially with eye movement.
- Loss of color vision
- Uhthoff's symptom (increased symptoms with exercise or increased body temperature)
- Pulfrich's phenomenon (altered perception of moving objects)
- May have had a preceding viral syndrome (upper respiratory, gastrointestinal, or other flulike symptoms).
- Other: focal neurologic symptoms (e.g., numbness or tingling in extremities).

■ **Clinical Manifestations**

- Decreased visual acuity with a relative afferent pupillary defect (RAPD).
- Decreased color vision and visual field defects.
- Swollen optic nerve [may have peripapillary flame-shaped hemorrhages (Plate 9)].
- Disc may appear normal in retrobulbar optic neuritis; usually seen in adults.
- Rarely, may see vitreous cells.

■ **Differential Diagnosis**

- Ischemic optic neuropathy (ION): sudden, painless loss of vision. Optic nerve swelling primarily pale. Visual field defects are usually inferior altitudinal. Usually no pain with ocular motility.
- Acute papilledema: disc edema is bilateral. Visual acuity and color vision are usually normal unless macular edema is present. Spontaneous venous pulsations absent. No pain with ocular

motility. No vitreous cells. Visual field testing often reveals enlarged blind spot.

- Severe systemic hypertension: bilateral disc edema with flame-shaped hemorrhages and cotton-wool spots. Blood pressure is elevated (Plate 8).
- Intracranial mass compressing the afferent visual pathway: Disc appears normal but there is loss of color vision with a positive RAPD. Neuroimaging of the brain reveals a mass.
- Orbital tumor compressing the optic nerve: optic nerve swelling (if present) would be unilateral. Proptosis or restriction of extraocular motility may be evident. Vitreous cells are not present.
- Toxic or metabolic optic neuropathy: progressive painless bilateral loss of vision secondary to malnutrition (vitamin B_1), alcohol, tobacco, pernicious anemia, or numerous toxins (e.g., heavy metals, ethambutol, isoniazid, chloroquine, digitalis). Optic discs appear pale, especially temporally.
- Leber's optic neuropathy: See discussion under differential diagnosis of papilledema above.

■ Diagnostic Evaluation

- Determine whether acute or gradual loss of vision is present. Inquire if there have been previous episodes or pain with ocular motility. Ask the patient's age.
- Perform ophthalmic examination including pupillary and color vision assessment. Perform dilated fundus examination to look for vitreous cells and swelling or hemorrhage in the retina or optic nerve.
- Visual field testing.
- Check blood pressure and perform neurologic examination looking for abnormalities.
- Consider blood tests such as CBC, ESR, RPR, FTA-ABS, and antinuclear antibody (ANA) if presentation is unusual such as no pain on eye movement or patient's age range is atypical.
- MRI with gadolinium of the brain and orbits for unusual cases and first episodes.

■ Treatment

- Observation if patient has a history of optic neuritis or MS.
- Intravenous steroids (e.g., methylprednisolone 250 mg IV every six hours) for 3 days followed by oral prednisone (e.g., 40–100 mg PO every day) if the patient is seen acutely and there is no previous history of optic neuritis or MS, and subsequent MRI of brain reveals at least one area of demyelination.
- Consider intravenous steroids to accelerate visual recovery in some patients.

- No oral prednisone as a primary treatment because this has been associated with an increased risk of recurrences.

■ Follow-up
- Every 1 to 3 months.
- Follow more closely and check IOP if on steroids.
- Neurology consult if CNS demyelination is seen on MRI.

Arteritic Ischemic Optic Neuropathy (Giant Cell Arteritis)

Ischemia to the optic nerve head as a result of giant cell arteritis (GCA). GCA is an autoimmune disease that affects arteries with an internal elastic lamina. GCA can result in myocardial infarction, stroke, and ocular complications.

■ Epidemiology
- Increased incidence with older age (more than 55 years)
- Usually occurs in whites (rare in blacks)

■ History
- Sudden, painless loss of vision without progression.
- Initially unilateral, but may rapidly become bilateral.
- May experience headache, jaw claudication (pain with chewing), or scalp tenderness.
- May have proximal muscle and joint pain (e.g., polymyalgia rheumatica), anorexia, weight loss, fever.
- Usually occurs in patients older than 50 years.

■ Clinical Manifestations
- Devastating loss of vision with an RAPD.
- Funduscopic examination reveals pale, swollen optic nerve (often associated with flame-shaped hemorrhages). As optic nerve edema resolves, optic atrophy ensues.
- Central retinal artery occlusion may occur.
- Visual field defects may occur revealing altitudinal or central visual loss.
- Palpated temporal artery may be tender and nonpulsatile.
- May acquire cranial nerve palsies (primarily CN VI).
- ESR may be very elevated.

■ Differential Diagnosis
- Nonarteritic ION. Usually patient is younger with less severe loss of vision. Usually do not have above symptoms of GCA; ESR is usually normal.

- Inflammatory optic neuritis (papillitis): Usually visual loss is less severe and less sudden. Pain is usually associated with eye movements. No symptoms of GCA. Associated with more hemorrhage of the optic disc. No vitreous cells. Usually younger persons affected.
- Central retinal vein occlusion (CRVO): severe loss of vision with associated RAPD. Optic nerve swelling is present as well as diffuse retinal hemorrhages (Blood and Thunder) extending to periphery.
- Compressive optic nerve tumor: slow progressive loss of visual acuity. No symptoms of GCA. Optic nerve slowly becomes pale.
- Central retinal artery occlusion (CRAO): sudden, severe, painless loss of vision associated with an RAPD. However, optic disc is not swollen. Retinal edema may be observed with a classic cherry-red spot in the fovea.

■ Diagnostic Evaluation

- Try to elicit above symptoms and ascertain the age of the patient, as older patients have a higher risk of developing GCA.
- Ocular examination: color vision testing and pupillary assessment to rule out RAPD. Dilated fundus examination for optic nerve evaluation and to rule out retinal causes of severe loss of vision.
- Stat ESR (Westergren). Upper limit of normal: men = age/2; women = (age + 10)/2.
- Temporal artery biopsy if symptoms or signs suspicious of GCA or ESR elevated.
- ESR may be normal (perform biopsy within 1 to 2 weeks of instituting steroid therapy).
- If biopsy is negative (at least a 2-cm section), a contralateral biopsy may be taken if a high clinical suspicion exists (some physicians prefer initial bilateral temporal artery biopsies because of skip areas and possible false negatives).

■ Treatment

- Once suspected, start intravenous steroids (e.g., methylprednisolone 250 mg IV every 6 hours for 12 doses) in the hospital. Switch to oral prednisone (e.g., 80–100 mg PO every day) after 12 doses.
- An oral antiulcer medication (e.g., ranitidine 150 mg PO twice per day) is often given concurrently with the steroid.
- Obtain temporal artery biopsy, often while the patient is still in the hospital.

- If biopsy is positive, continue oral prednisone. Steroid may be slowly tapered over 3 to 12 months as ESR declines or symptoms improve. Patient's internist should manage complications of steroid therapy, but an ophthalmologist should adjust and taper the steroid level based on clinical findings and the ESR.
- Discontinue steroids after obtaining negative biopsies on adequate specimens.

■ Follow-up

- Evaluate and treat emergently if GCA suspected.
- After diagnosis confirmed by biopsy, initial steroid dosage is continued for 4 weeks until symptoms improve or ESR decreases.
- Taper steroid very slowly over 3 to 12 months.
- Decrease dosage monthly as symptoms reverse or ESR decreases.
- Check ESR monthly with each dosage change.
  - If symptoms return or ESR elevates, steroid dose must be increased.
  - Use minimal steroid dose to achieve desired result.

Nonarteritic Ischemic Optic Neuropathy

Ischemia of the optic nerve head due to compromise of the posterior ciliary vessels.

■ History

- Sudden moderate, nonprogressive loss of vision; painless
- Initially unilateral but may become bilateral

■ Clinical Manifestations

- RAPD and decreased color vision
- Optic disc with flame-shaped hemorrhages and often pale swelling involving only one sector
- Optic atrophy after edema resolves (Plate 5)
- Altitudinal or central visual field defect
- Normal ESR

■ Risk Factors

- Often associated with hypertension, diabetes, arteriosclerosis
- Patients usually 40 to 60 years old

■ Differential Diagnosis

- See Arteritic Ischemic Optic Neuropathy above.

■ Diagnostic Evaluation
- Ask about above symptoms of GCA. Determining age is very important (usually occurs in 40- to 60-year-olds).
- Ocular examination: evaluate pupils for RAPD and check color vision with color plates. Dilated fundus examination to evaluate the optic nerve and to rule out retinal causes of severe visual loss.

■ Treatment/Follow-up
- Observation
- Follow-up in 1 month

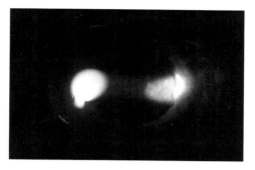

Plate 1 • Slit beam focused on the anterior chamber demonstrating inflammatory cells and flare (leaking protein from vasculature) as seen in uveitis and other inflammatory conditions. *(Image courtesy of Anton Drew, Queen Elizabeth Hospital, Woodville South, Australia.)*

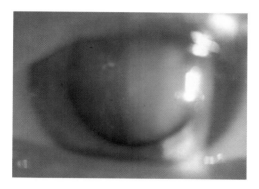

Plate 2 • Pigment cells in the vitreous are seen here by focusing the slit beam just posterior to the lens. The presence of vitreous pigmented cells necessitates ruling out a rhegmatogenous retinal detachment.

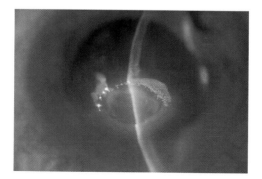

Plate 3 • Corneal ulcers appear as white and opaque lesions. This ulcer has no overlying epithelium, and surrounding corneal stromal edema is often present.

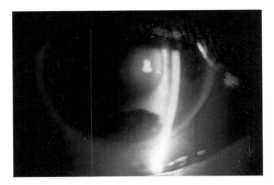

Plate 4 • A hyphema is the presence of blood in the anterior chamber. It may be layered, or it may be seen as a clot (as shown here) or as red blood cells floating in the anterior chamber (microhyphema). Hyphemas usually result from blunt trauma but may occur in association with neovascularization of the iris (rubeosis).

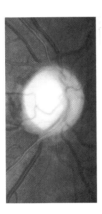

Plate 5 • Optic atrophy results from degeneration of nerve fibers at the optic nerve head and demonstrates pallor. This can occur in chronic disc edema. A relative afferent pupillary defect is usually present.

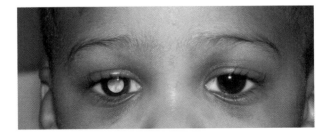

Plate 6 • Leukocoria. A lesion in the optical media or retina results in loss of the normal red reflex. *(Image courtesy of Dr. Janice Lasky, Children's Memorial Hospital, Chicago, Illinois.)*

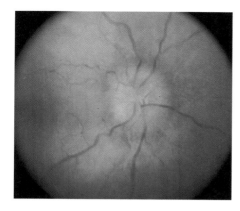

Plate 7 • Disc edema secondary to increased intracranial hypertension demonstrates an elevated disc with a hyperemic neuro-retinal rim and dilated capillaries.

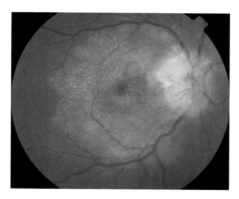

Plate 8 • Disc edema secondary to uncontrolled hypertension. Note the blurred disc margins and hemorrhages and evidence of hypertensive retinopathy. Leaking lipids travel in Henle's layer toward the macula forming a "macular star."

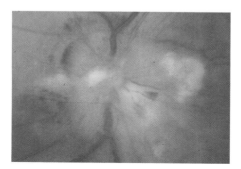

Plate 9 • Disc edema secondary to malignant hypertension, optic neuritis, or ischemic optic neuropathy demonstrates hemorrhagic disc swelling with exudates and cotton-wool spots surrounding the optic nerve. The disc margin is very blurred.

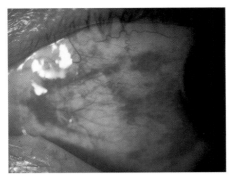

Plate 10 • A subconjunctival hemorrhage appears as bright red areas overlying the sclera, which usually clear within 2 weeks.

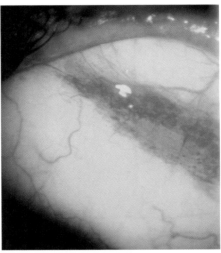

Plate 11 • Kaposi's sarcoma of the conjunctiva (or lids and skin) is usually seen in AIDS patients. These are highly vascular lesions and when present in the conjunctiva may be mistaken for a subconjunctival hemorrhage. (Photo originally from the collection of Dr. Dale Henderly [deceased], and provided courtesy of Dr. Gary Lissner, Department of Ophthalmology, Northwestern University Feinberg School of Medicine, Chicago, Illinois.)

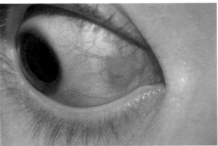

Plate 12 • Deep inflamed vessels of scleritis. These vessels do not move with manipulation and do not blanch with topical phenylephrine (as do vessels in episcleritis).

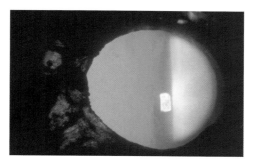

Plate 13 • Transillumination defects in iris atrophy seen by retroillumination. In pigment dispersion syndrome these defects would be present more in the peripheral iris and would appear as spokelike.

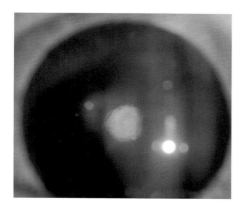

Plate 14 • A posterior subcapsular cataract is seen as a rough plaque on the posterior aspect of the lens.

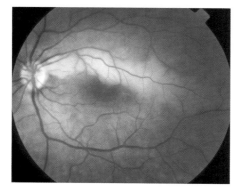

Plate 15 • Branch retinal artery occlusion (BRAO) of the superior temporal arcade revealing edematous opacification of the retina as a result of ischemia. A cherry-red spot is seen in the fovea in a central retinal artery occlusion (CRAO) because the orange reflex from the intact choroidal vasculature beneath the intact fovea stands out in contrast to the surrounding opaque neural retina.

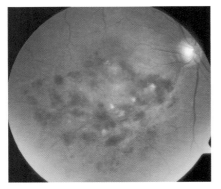

Plate 16 • Branch retinal vein occlusion (BRVO) of the inferior temporal arcade with typical dot-and-blot hemorrhages ("blood and thunder").

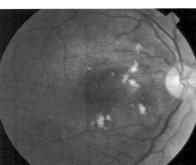

Plate 17 • Cotton-wool spots are white fluffy lesions with indistinct borders found at the edges of microinfarcts in the nerve fiber layer, usually close to the optic nerve where the nerve fiber layer is thickest. They are most commonly seen in hypertensive retinopathy but occur in other vascular occlusive diseases (e.g., diabetes and BRVO/CRVO).

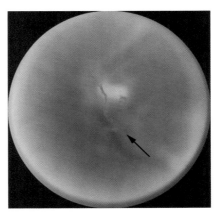

Plate 18 • A Weiss ring may be seen in cases of a posterior vitreous detachment. The normal vitreous attaches to the margins of the optic disc and separates during a posterior vitreous detachment. The ring usually folds on itself assuming various shapes. It is best viewed when observing the optic nerve at the slit lamp with high-power magnification and pulling back slowly on the joystick. Here, it is seen anterior and inferior to the optic nerve.

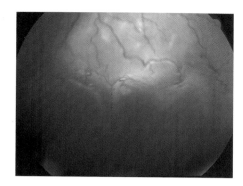

Plate 19 • A rhegmatogenous retinal detachment (RRD) often appears as a pinkish grey membrane with a corrugated appearance. An RD often undulates with eye movements (especially with recent RDs).

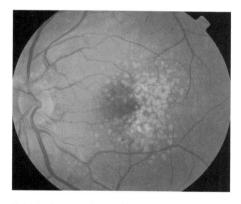

Plate 20 • Multiple discrete subretinal lesions are called drusen. Age-related macular degeneration (AMD) is present when drusen in the macula are associated with decreased vision not explained by another process (dry AMD).

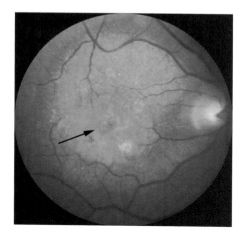

Plate 21 • Wet age-related macular degeneration presents with a subretinal hemorrhage secondary to a choroidal neovascular membrane.

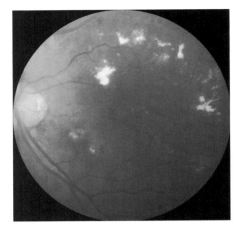

Plate 22 • Background diabetic retinopathy often demonstrates microaneurysms and hard exudates (yellow glistening bodies) on the posterior pole.

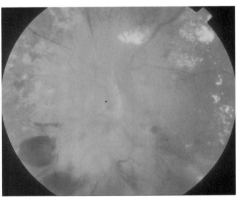

Plate 23 • Proliferative diabetic retinopathy results in neovascularization of the retina or disc and dot-and-blot retinal hemorrhages. A preretinal hemorrhage is evident inferiorly here from rupture of the neovascular vessels.

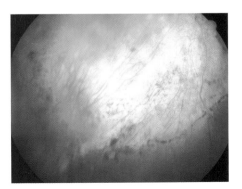

Plate 24 • A whitish area of the retina, associated with hemorrhage is typically seen in cytomegalovirus (CMV) retinitis. There is usually an associated mild vitritis.

7

Cornea and External Ocular Diseases

P. Oat Sinchai, MD and Thomas E. Bournias, MD

Blepharitis/Meibomianitis

Inflammation of the eyelid margins

■ Pathogenesis

- Three main causes of blepharitis
  - Staphylococcal: overgrowth of normal skin/eyelid flora with immunologic hypersensitivity reaction to their antigens
  - Meibomian gland dysfunction: results in lipid tear deficiency, which in turn results in tear film instability and increased tear film evaporation
  - Seborrheic: abnormal oily skin with increased and thickened meibomian gland secretions

■ History

- Burning, itching, foreign body sensation
- Blurry vision
- Red eye/eyelids; eyelid crusting
- Recurrent chalazia

■ Clinical Manifestations

- Bulbar and tarsal conjunctival injection.
- Inflamed eyelid margin with telangiectatic vessels, and hard or oily crusting around lashes.
- Thickened, turbid meibomian gland secretions.
- Decreased tear meniscus, often with foam along lower eyelid margin.
- Superficial punctate keratitis (SPK) in the inferior cornea that stains with fluorescein.
- Marginal epithelial/subepithelial infiltrates.
- Corneal scarring/pannus and phlyctenules.
- Acne rosacea may be present.

■ Risk Factors

- Acne rosacea
- Oral retinoid therapy

■ Differential Diagnosis

- Conjunctivitis: Allergic: associated with watery/mucoid discharge, itching; Viral: associated with watery discharge and possible palpable preauricular node; Bacterial: associated with purulent discharge. (See Chapter 3, Red Eye p. 28 Table 3-1.)
- Aqueous tear deficiency (dry eye syndrome): similar symptoms as blepharitis, but no lid margin or meibomian gland abnormalities; foam/debris in tear film; punctate epithelial erosions in interpalpebral space that stain with fluorescein; abnormal Schirmer's test (tear flow test).
- Sebaceous gland carcinoma: unilateral eyelid margin inflammation/irregularity with loss of eyelashes (rarely, unilateral, intractable blepharitis is the only manifestation of sebaceous cell carcinoma).

■ Diagnostic Evaluation

- History and slit lamp examination with attention to eyelid margin/lashes/meibomian gland orifices/conjunctiva for the findings mentioned above. May note rapid tear film breakup time with fluorescein and decreased tear film meniscus.

■ Treatment

- Eyelid hygiene:
  - Apply warm compresses to eyelids for a few minutes to liquefy thickened meibomian gland secretions and soften crusting on eyelid margins.
  - Massage eyelids to express plugged/retained meibomian gland secretions.
  - Clean eyelid margin/lashes with a cotton-tipped applicator with warm water and/or diluted baby shampoo every night.
  - Administer topical antibiotic ointment (e.g., erythromycin or bacitracin) to the eyelids every night to decrease staphylococcal colonization of eyelids.
- May consider short course of topical steroid (e.g., loteprednol etabonate 0.5% or prednisolone acetate 1%, one drop four times per day) for patients with severe inflammation, corneal infiltrates, or neovascularization.
- Oral tetracycline (250 mg PO four times per day) or oral doxycycline (50–100 mg PO daily or twice daily) for 2 to 6 weeks. Some patients with chronic disease may require therapy for longer than six weeks.
- Artificial tears (e.g., Refresh Tears, Genteal, or Systane) when necessary if associated with dry eye.
- Consider cyclosporine emulsion (e.g., Restasis, one drop twice per day) if associated with dry eyes.

- Manage any existing chalazia with warm compresses or incision and drainage.
- Manage any existing ocular rosacea with systemic tetracyclines, lid hygiene, or metronidazole gel 0.75% to affected facial areas.

Note: Tetracycline is contraindicated during pregnancy, in women who are nursing, and in patients with known hypersensitivity.

Dry Eye Syndrome

Tear film distortion due to tear deficiency or excessive tear evaporation causing damage to the interpalpebral ocular surface and associated with symptoms of ocular discomfort. It results from a localized immune-mediated inflammatory response affecting both the lacrimal gland and the ocular surface.

■ Pathogenesis

- Aqueous tear deficiency due to lacrimal gland dysfunction: causes include congenital, inflammatory (Sjögren's syndrome, rheumatoid arthritis), traumatic, anticholinergic medications, decreased corneal sensation [following photorefractive keratectomy (PRK) or laser-assisted in situ keratomileusis (LASIK)].
- Mucin tear deficiency due to goblet cell dysfunction: causes include vitamin A deficiency, chemical burn, cicatricial pemphigoid, Stevens-Johnson syndrome, and trachoma.
- Lipid tear deficiency due to meibomian gland dysfunction (see Blepharitis above).

■ Epidemiology

- Affects 10% to 15% of adults

■ History

- Bilateral foreign body/scratchy sensation, burning, tearing.
- Blurred vision.
- Symptoms tend to worsen toward the end of the day, with prolonged use of the eyes, or with exposure to dry or windy conditions.

■ Clinical Manifestations

- Tear film meniscus less than 1 mm and/or increased tear breakup time
- Conjunctival injection; irregular corneal surface and corneal SPK, which stain with fluorescein

- Mucous plaques and filaments (core of mucus covered by strands of epithelial cells attached to the surface of the cornea)
- Marginal or paracentral thinning of the cornea

■ Risk Factors
- Contact lens wearers often have decreased tear production, likely due to decreased corneal sensation.
- Women, especially postmenopausal (appears associated with decreased androgen).
- Age greater than 60.
- Birth control pills and other medications (e.g., antihistamines, anticholinergics).

■ Differential Diagnosis
- Conjunctivitis (see pp. 83–84)
- Blepharitis: will have the characteristic lid margin findings in blepharitis
- Exposure keratopathy: eyelid abnormality often resulting from seventh-nerve palsy, trauma, or ectropion/entropion

■ Diagnostic Evaluation
- History and physical examination with attention to determining the inciting cause.
- Slit lamp examination: Examine tear meniscus and tear break-up time with fluorescein stain. Examine surface of cornea and conjunctiva with rose bengal and lissamine stains.
- Schirmer's test (anesthetized): to detect decreased aqueous tear production (normally 10 mm or more).

■ Treatment
- Artificial tears (e.g., Refresh Tears, Genteal, Systane), gels, or ointments (preferably preservative free if used more than four times per day).
- Changing/discontinuing use of any medications that decrease tear production (diuretics, antihistamines, anticholinergics, psychotropics).
- Punctal occlusion with plugs (temporary) or cautery (permanent).
- Topical cyclosporine emulsion (e.g., Restasis, one drop twice per day): modulates inflammatory response (by inhibiting activated T lymphocytes responsible for destruction of the lacrimal gland, thereby improving lacrimal secretion).
- Short course of topical steroids (e.g., loteprednol etabonate 0.5% or prednisolone acetate 1%, one drop four times per day) for

quicker suppression of inflammatory component. Consider short course of topical steroids immediately before or at the time of initiation of cyclosporine emulsion because cyclosporine may take 1 to 3 months or more before symptoms improve.

- Remove mucus strands or filaments if present with jewelers forceps.
- Tarsorrhaphy for severe dry eye if above modalities are without relief.
- Address contributing disorders such as blepharitis (see blepharitis treatment, pp. 80–81).
- Refer to internist if symptoms are suggestive of collagen vascular disease (e.g., dry mouth, joint pain, or rash).

■ Follow-up
- Days to months depending on severity of disease

Conjunctivitis

Inflammation of the conjunctiva with many etiologic factors, including bacterial [especially *Staphylococcus* or *Neisseria* if hyperacute (less than 24 hours)], viral (typically adenovirus), and allergic (IgE mediated). See Table 3-1 for distinguishing signs/symptoms.

■ History
- Sudden onset of redness with discharge
- Itching (allergic)
- Photophobia (viral)

■ Clinical Manifestations
- Conjunctival hyperemia/chemosis
- Bacterial: purulent discharge, papillary reaction of the palpebral conjunctiva
- Viral: watery discharge, follicular conjunctival reaction, eyelid edema, and palpable preauricular node
- Allergic: watery/mucoid discharge, papillary conjunctival reaction

■ Risk Factors
- Bacterial: contact lens overuse.
- Viral: recent or associated upper respiratory tract infection. Contact with a person with viral conjunctivitis or upper respiratory tract infection.
- Allergic: atopy, asthma, and/or seasonal allergies.

■ **Differential Diagnosis**

- See Table 3-1 (p. 28) to distinguish:
  - Bacterial conjunctivitis
  - Viral conjunctivitis
  - Allergic conjunctivitis
- Blepharoconjunctivitis: associated with lid margin and conjunctival hyperemia, debris in tear film, punctate corneal epithelial erosions, meibomian gland plugging

■ **Diagnostic Evaluation**

- History and slit lamp examination with attention to the palpebral conjunctiva to evaluate papillary/follicular reaction.
- Palpate for preauricular lymph nodes.

■ **Treatment**

- Bacterial:
  - Broad-spectrum topical antibiotics (e.g., tobramycin, gatifloxacin, or moxifloxacin, one drop four times per day)
  - Frequent irrigation and systemic ceftriaxone (1 gram IM) or ciprofloxacin (500 mg PO, single dose) for gonococcal (*Neisseria gonorrhoeae*) conjunctivitis
- Viral
  - Cool compresses/artificial tears
  - Frequent hand washing to prevent transmission to other people or to the uninvolved eye
- Allergic
  - Cool compresses/artificial tears
  - Topical antihistamine and/or mast cell stabilizer (e.g., ketotifen fumarate, epinastine hydrochloride, olopatadine hydrochloride, each one drop twice per day)
  - Topical nonsteroidal anti-inflammatory drugs (NSAIDs) (e.g., ketorolac tromethamine, one drop 2–4 times per day)
  - Oral antihistamine if itching persists (e.g., loratadine, 10 mg PO every day)

■ **Follow-up**

- Bacterial: 1 to 7 days, depending on severity
- Viral and allergic: 1 to 4 weeks, depending on severity

Subconjunctival Hemorrhage

Ruptured subconjunctival blood vessel secondary to trauma, Valsalva maneuver (vomiting, coughing, sneezing, straining, etc.), hypertension, bleeding disorder, or anticoagulation (Plate 10). May also be idiopathic.

■ **History**

- Sudden onset of bright red blood underneath the conjunctiva
- Usually asymptomatic, but may have mild irritation
- History of trauma, vomiting, coughing, or other forms of Valsalva maneuver

■ **Clinical Manifestations**

- Hemorrhage underneath the conjunctiva, usually sectorial; occasionally raises up the conjunctiva
- May be very bright red and completely obscure view of the sclera
- Becomes yellow as it resolves over 2 to 3 weeks

■ **Differential Diagnosis**

- Kaposi's sarcoma: slightly elevated red or purplish vascular subconjunctival lesion often associated with acquired immunodeficiency syndrome (AIDS) (Plate 11).
- Lymphoma: pink mobile conjunctival or subconjunctival lesion, which may bleed and cause a subconjunctival hemorrhage. Patients are often older than 50 years or immunosuppressed.

■ **Diagnostic Evaluation**

- Ascertain if there is a history of a bleeding disorder or use of anticoagulation medication (e.g., warfarin, aspirin). Ask if there had been Valsalva maneuvers or heavy lifting, straining, or coughing. Determine if there had been any recent trauma or eye rubbing.
- For those with a history of trauma, must rule out intraocular damage and/or ruptured globe with slit lamp examination, tonometry, and dilated fundus examination.
- Check blood pressure if history cannot explain hemorrhage and there is no known previous history of hypertension.
- For recurrent hemorrhages, check CBC (to rule out leukemia) and platelets, bleeding time, prothrombin time/international normalized ratio, partial thromboplastin time, protein C and S.

■ **Treatment**

- Reassurance: patients should be told that the hemorrhage might enlarge and/or change color (red to yellow to green) as it resolves.
- No therapy necessary; usually resolves within 2 to 3 weeks.
- Patients with mild irritation may take artificial tears as needed.
- Avoid elective use of oral aspirin and NSAIDs.
- Refer to internist if hypertension or abnormal blood tests found or if no apparent cause found for recurrent hemorrhages.

■ **Follow-up**

• As needed or if not resolved after 2 to 3 weeks

Pinguecula/Pterygium

Elastoid degeneration of the nasal and/or temporal bulbar conjunctival collagen secondary to ultraviolet exposure, dryness, inflammation, wind, and dust. A pterygium is a wing-shaped fibrovascular fold of conjunctiva invading the superficial cornea (Figure 7-1). A pterygium is almost always preceded and accompanied by pinguecula, but it is not known why some patients develop pterygia whereas others have only pinguecula.

■ **Epidemiology**

• The prevalence of pterygia increases toward the equator.

■ **History**

• Recurrent inflammation, irritation, and redness.
• Pterygium may cause decreased vision and/or astigmatism, depending on its size.
• May be asymptomatic.

■ **Clinical Manifestations**

• Pinguecula: a flat or raised yellow-white lesion occurring on the nasal and/or temporal bulbar conjunctiva near the limbus in the interpalpebral zone. Does not involve the cornea.

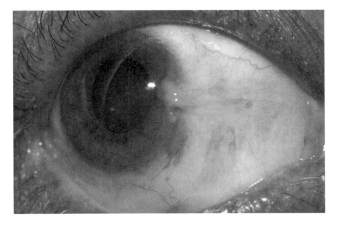

Figure 7-1 • Pterygium.

- Pterygium: a wing-shaped fibrovascular fold of conjunctiva invading the superficial cornea (see Figure 7-1).
  -**Stocker's line:** pigmented iron line seen in front of a pterygium on the cornea

■ Differential Diagnosis

- Nodular episcleritis and scleritis (Plate 12): may appear similar to pinguecula, but the symptoms are typically more painful and irritating (see episcleritis and scleritis, pp. 88–92)
- Corneal pannus: may mimic pterygia, but are typically more vascular and often can be linked to an underlying problem (e.g., contact lens overuse, blepharitis, trachoma, ocular rosacea)
- Conjunctival epithelial neoplasia: are not in a wing-shaped formation, are white lesions, and often elevated and vascularized

■ Diagnostic Evaluation

- History and slit lamp examination to evaluate the lesion and its relationship to the cornea

■ Treatment

- Artificial tears/gel/ointment
- Topical NSAIDs (e.g., ketorolac tromethamine, one drop 2–4 times per day) or steroids (e.g., prednisolone acetate 1% or loteprednol etabonate 0.5%, one drop four times per day) for more severe cases
- Eyewear to protect from the elements including sun and wind
- Vasoconstriction (e.g., tetrahydrozoline, one drop PRN) on a limited basis
- Excision:
  -Pinguecula: for cosmesis, chronic inflammation, or interfering with contact lens wear
  -Pterygium: for irritation, induced astigmatism, or threatening the visual axis

  Note: Pterygium often recur after surgical excision. In this case, use of antimetabolites (e.g., 5-fluorouracil), autografts, or human amniotic membrane allografts reduce the recurrence rate.

■ Follow-up

- Weeks to years, depending on severity and use of topical steroids.
- More frequently when using topical steroids to monitor inflammation and IOP.
- Taper steroids when inflammation subsides.

Episcleritis

A temporary, self-limited, usually benign inflammation of the episcleral resulting in a sectorial engorgement of blood vessels. Pathophysiology is not known, with most cases being idiopathic.

■ Etiology

- Idiopathic (most common)
- Connective tissue disease:
  -Systemic lupus erythematosus, rheumatoid arthritis, polyarteritis nodosa
  -Ankylosing spondylitis, Wegener's granulomatosis
- Infection
  -Herpes simplex virus (HSV), herpes zoster virus (HZV)
  -Syphilis
  -Lyme, tuberculosis, Reiter's syndrome
- Inflammatory conditions
  -Inflammatory bowel disease, sarcoidosis
- Rosacea, atopy
- Following ocular surgery
- Others: thyroid disease, gout

■ History

- Acute unilateral or bilateral red eye, usually asymptomatic, but may have mild tenderness
- No discharge; does not affect vision

■ Clinical Manifestations

- Two types:
  -Simple: sectorial or diffuse inflammation with radially directed vessels
  -Nodular: localized inflamed mobile nodule
- Normal vision but may have mild to moderate tenderness
- Rarely, some patients may have a small peripheral corneal opacity bordering the inflammation.

■ Differential Diagnosis

- Scleritis: severe pain; deeper inflammation; sclera may have violet hue in natural lighting. Dilated vessels have a criss-cross pattern and do not blanch with topical 2.5% phenylephrine hydrochloride (Neo-Synephrine).
- Conjunctivitis: more irritation and/or pain; may have discharge and tarsal conjunctival papillae or follicles.

■ Diagnostic Evaluation

- History and slit lamp examination to localize the inflammation to the episcleral tissue:
  - Episcleritis will demonstrate superficial injection of vessels in a radial pattern with a bright red hue.
  - After application of topical proparacaine, the vessels can be moved with a cotton-tipped applicator. They also blanch after 15 minutes with topical phenylephrine 2.5%.

■ Treatment

- Reassurance: will not affect vision and generally resolves spontaneously.
- Mild pain/irritation can be managed with lubrication or topical/oral NSAIDs. Topical steroids (e.g., prednisone acetate 1%, one drop four times per day) may be used judiciously in patients whose disease is severe or is not responsive to standard therapy.
- Multiple recurrences, bilateral involvement, or appropriate history should trigger a workup for etiologies listed above. Tests include ESR, FTA-ABS, RPR, ANA, ANCA, rheumatoid factor, and serum uric acid level.

■ Follow-up

- One week to a few months depending on the severity of disease.
- Check weekly if on topical steroids until symptoms resolve (watch for elevated IOP).

Scleritis

Immune-mediated or infectious vasculitis of the sclera. Classified by location and characteristics of inflammation. May be associated with an underlying systemic immunologic disease (Plate 12).

■ Etiology

See discussion of etiology for episcleritis above.

■ History

- Gradual onset of severe, deep, aching eye pain, which may worsen at night and awaken the patient from sleep.
- Eye may be tender to palpation, and pain is often referred to the head or face.
- Eye slowly becomes red with progressive decrease in vision.
- Minimal symptoms in scleromalacia perforans.

■ Clinical Manifestations
- The inflammation casts a violet hue, more easily seen in natural lighting.
- The deep inflamed vessels have a criss-cross pattern and cannot be moved by manipulation (Plate 12).
- Scleral and episcleral edema.

Anterior Scleritis
- Diffuse anterior scleritis: area of scleral injection and edema; may involve only a portion of or all of the anterior segment
- Nodular anterior scleritis: dark red/violet, fixed scleral nodule, separate from the overlying episclera
- Necrotizing scleritis: most destructive form of scleritis. A significant number of patients suffer loss of vision and/or develop ocular and systemic disease. Sometimes associated with inflammation.

NECROTIZING SCLERITIS WITH INFLAMMATION
- Initially presents as a localized area of inflammation with severe pain.
- If left untreated, disease may spread with severe loss of sclera and adjacent tissue until the entire anterior segment is affected.
- The sclera thins and the underlying choroid becomes visible (casts a blue/gray hue).
- High rate of association with systemic inflammatory disease.

NECROTIZING SCLERITIS WITHOUT INFLAMMATION (SCLEROMALACIA PERFORANS)
- Usually painless with very mild signs of inflammation.
- The sclera thins and the underlying choroid becomes visible (casts a blue/gray hue).
- A staphyloma or outpouching of the sclera may develop if IOP is high.
- Often seen in patients with chronic rheumatoid arthritis.

Posterior Scleritis
- May occur by itself or in association with anterior scleritis.
- Presents with pain, proptosis, visual loss, and possibly restricted ocular motility.
- Other possible sequelae include retraction of lower eyelid in upgaze, choroidal folds, exudative retinal detachment, papilledema, and angle-closure glaucoma.
- Rapid-onset hyperopia.
- Referred pain to other parts of the head/face.

- Demonstration of thickened posterior sclera by echography, CT, or MRI may be helpful in establishing the diagnosis (T-sign).
- Often no related disease can be found in patients with posterior scleritis.

■ Differential Diagnosis

- Episcleritis: less pain with more acute onset, more of a bright red hue with vessels in a radial pattern. Vessels are not deep and can be localized to the episclera with a cotton-tipped applicator. Vessels blanch with topical phenylephrine 2.5%

■ Diagnostic Evaluation

- History and complete eye examination to evaluate for signs listed above.
- Ultrasound, CT/MRI of the orbits may demonstrate thickened posterior sclera (in posterior scleritis).
- Complete physical examination with attention to the joints, skin, cardiovascular and respiratory systems (best done in conjunction with a rheumatologist or other internist).
- Initial screening tests may include CBC w/differential, ESR, C-reactive protein, ANA, anti-DNA antibody, rheumatoid factor, ANCA, urinalysis, serum uric acid, syphilis serology, chest x-ray, angiotensin-converting enzyme (ACE) level, and lysozyme to evaluate for systemic autoimmune or infectious disease.

■ Treatment

- Oral NSAIDs (e.g., ibuprofen 400–800 mg PO 2 to 4 times per day) for 1 to 3 weeks. (NSAIDs are not helpful for necrotizing scleritis.)
- If no improvement on oral NSAIDs, try systemic steroids (e.g., prednisone 60–100 mg/day) for 2 to 3 weeks, followed by tapering.
- Concurrent antacid (e.g., ranitidine 150 mg PO two times per day) while patient is on systemic steroids/NSAIDs.
- Consider immunosuppressive therapy (e.g., methotrexate, cyclosporine) if steroids ineffective.
- Topical steroids are minimally effective (and are contraindicated in necrotizing scleritis because of the risk of scleral thinning and perforation).
- For scleromalacia perforans: judicious lubrication is warranted, and consideration for scleral reinforcement surgery (such as with Tutoplast) with a graft may be necessary if there is significant risk of perforation.

■ Follow-up
• Days to months depending on the severity of disease and amount of scleral thinning present.

Recurrent Corneal Erosion

Sudden recurrent sharp pain lasting for seconds to minutes resulting from the eyelid's pulling off areas of epithelium. This is a result of poor adhesion of the corneal epithelium to its underlying basement membrane and Bowman's layer resulting in recurrent epithelial defects/erosions. Usually patients either have an underlying corneal epithelial basement membrane dystrophy or have a history of a sudden shearing/abrading injury to their eye causing an epithelial defect that does not heal properly (often not clinically evident). Symptoms suddenly recur, especially upon awakening in the morning, without any obvious cause and resolve spontaneously, with recurrences occurring periodically.

■ History
• Sudden onset of eye pain, usually at night or upon waking, when eyelids are opened.
• Associated with redness, photophobia, and tearing, with symptoms lasting seconds to hours.
• Often there is a history of injury with subsequent corneal abrasion to the involved eye.

■ Clinical Manifestations
• May have a frank epithelial defect, loose but intact epithelium, edematous corneal epithelium, and/or only subtle corneal abnormalities with mild to minimal stain with fluorescein dye.
• Patients' symptoms often seem out of proportion to clinical findings because epithelial damage may resolve within hours.
• More severe episodes may involve eyelid edema and decreased vision.
• Fingerprint pattern or maplike lines may be seen in both corneas if map-dot-fingerprint dystrophy is present.

■ Risk Factors
• Previous ocular trauma/corneal abrasion
• Corneal epithelial basement membrane dystrophy
• Corneal dystrophies of the stroma and Bowman's layer

- Previous eye surgery including corneal transplantation and keratorefractive (e.g., LASIK or PRK)

■ Differential Diagnosis

- Herpes simplex keratitis: may have intermittent episodes of unilateral pain with characteristic dendritic keratitis, which stains with fluorescein. May have typical skin lesions (vesicles) and intraocular involvement (such as uveitis or retinitis).

■ Diagnostic Evaluation

- Ascertain if there is history of recent trauma/corneal abrasion.
- Slit lamp examination: erosions will stain with fluorescein while subtle areas of loosely adherent epithelium can be identified by gently manipulating the epithelium with a cotton-tipped applicator after placing a drop of topical anesthetic in the eye. Corneal epithelial dots or microcysts may be seen.

■ Treatment

- Artificial tears and/or antibiotic ointment at least three to four times per day. Lubrication may need to be continued for 3 to 6 months to prevent recurrence.
- Hypertonic saline solution (e.g., Muro 128, 5% NaCl, one drop four times per day): temporarily produces an osmotic gradient, drawing fluid from the epithelium, improving its adherence to the underlying basement membrane.
- Bandage contact lens: reduces pain and protects the epithelium from further damage. Use with topical broad-spectrum antibiotics to reduce the possibility of secondary infection.
- Anterior stromal micropuncture: multiple superficial punctures using a bent 27-gauge needle to the involved area to improve adhesion between the epithelium and its basement membrane.
  -Use with caution in visual axis.
- Epithelial debridement: after applying topical anesthetic, debride loose epithelium with a surgical sponge, spatula, or blade. Antibiotic ointment, cycloplegic drops, and/or bandage contact lenses are used until reepithelialization occurs.
- PRK: creates a large, shallow zone of ablation, which seems to improve adhesion between the epithelium and basement membrane. Especially successful in patients with corneal dystrophies.

■ Follow-up

- Days to weeks depending on severity of disease
- Every 1 to 2 days until epithelium healed

Herpes Simplex Virus

HSV type 1 is a common cause of ocular disease that is usually acquired early in life as a result of direct contact with active lesions; however, it often results from exposure to viral organisms shed asymptomatically. HSV type 1 primarily causes orofacial and ocular infection. HSV type 2 typically causes genital infection but may sometimes cause ocular infection. Primary HSV-1 infection typically occurs on skin or mucosal surfaces innervated by cranial nerve (CN) V, and spreads via sensory nerve axons to become latent in the trigeminal ganglia. Reactivation of HSV may follow any of the three branches of CN V.

■ Epidemiology

- Most people older than 60 years have HSV latent in their trigeminal ganglia at biopsy.
- Approximately one third of the world population suffers from recurrent infection.

■ History

- Typically unilateral foreign body sensation, photophobia, red eye.
- Blurred vision.
- Occasionally, there is a history of previous episodes.

■ Clinical Manifestations (See Table 7-1)

- Blepharoconjunctivitis: typically unilateral (10% bilateral), follicular conjunctival inflammation with vesicles on the skin or lid margin and palpable preauricular lymph node
- Epithelial keratitis: punctate erosions may coalesce into a dendritic ulcer with terminal bulbs at the end of each branch (see Figure 4-1, p. 36); other findings include corneal stromal edema, subepithelial white blood cell infiltration, conjunctival injection, ciliary flush, and decreased corneal sensitivity
- Stromal keratitis:
  - Interstitial (nonnecrotizing): interstitial stromal haze and edema with intact epithelium
  - Disciform (nonnecrotizing): stromal and epithelial edema in an oval distribution with underlying keratic precipitates (KP), minimal anterior chamber reaction, and intact epithelium
  - Necrotizing: severe, rapidly progressive suppurative stromal infiltrate with overlying epithelial ulcer; associated stromal thinning, neovascularization, or iritis/hypopyon
- Iridocyclitis: granulomatous or nongranulomatous; elevated IOP secondary to trabeculitis (inflammation of the trabecular meshwork)
- Rarely retinitis

■ TABLE 7-1 Differentiating Features of HSV and HZV		
	HSV	**HZV**
Virus	*Herpes-Simplex-1*	*Varicella-Zoster*
dendritic morphology	dendrite with terminal bulbs	pseudodendrite
dermatomal distribution	incomplete	complete
skin scarring	rare	frequent
pain	less	more
postherpetic neuralgia	rare	common
bilateral involvement	rare	never

■ Differential Diagnosis (of dendrite-appearing corneal lesions)

- Herpes zoster virus (HZV): skin lesions/vesicles follow a dermatomal pattern, do not cross the midline, and eventually crust over. Pseudodendrites have a "stuck-on" appearance and stain poorly with fluorescein. The pseudodendrites do not have terminal bulbs but are raised mucous plaques.
- *Acanthamoeba:* Patients usually have a history of contact lens wear or homemade saline solution. Often, severe pain is out of proportion to inflammation. Pseudodendrites are similar to HZV; no skin involvement.
- Recurrent corneal erosion: the healing erosion may have the appearance of a dendrite. The patient often has a history of corneal abrasion in the involved eye.
- Contact lens wear: epithelial defects are not dendritic and do not stain as strongly as HSV. There is often micropannus of the cornea (especially superiorly), but no skin involvement.

■ Diagnostic Evaluation

- Ascertain if there is a history of episodes of previous nasal, oral, or genital sores.
- Examine skin and lids for vesicles.
- Perform slit lamp examination to determine if there is ocular involvement and check IOP.
- Test corneal sensation with a tiny wisp of cotton from a cotton-tipped applicator before using anesthetic drops (corneal sensation often reduced in HSV).
- In complicated cases, tissue culture and/or HSV antigen detection techniques, including Papanicolaou's stain and enzyme-linked immunosorbent assay may be helpful.

■ Treatment
- Primary ocular HSV infection is a self-limited condition.
- Oral antiviral therapy (e.g., acyclovir 600–800 mg PO five times per day or famciclovir 500 mg PO three times per day) for 7 to 14 days speeds resolution of signs and symptoms, and is used long term to reduce the rate of recurrence.
- Topical trifluridine (e.g., Viroptic) or vidarabine five times per day for 10 to 14 days (avoid prolonged use to prevent corneal toxicity) for eyelid margin involvement, conjunctivitis, or corneal epithelial involvement.
- Topical steroids are contraindicated in active epithelial keratitis but are used in conjunction with topical antiviral drops for stromal keratitis.
- Penetrating keratoplasty for severe inactive corneal scars that are visually significant.

■ Follow-up
- Every few days, until condition improves

Varicella-Zoster Virus

Varicella-zoster virus (or HZV) causes a primary infection (chickenpox) in direct contact with skin lesions or respiratory secretions. The virus becomes latent in sensory ganglia and may reactivate later causing zoster/shingles. Involvement with varicella-zoster virus of the ophthalmic division of the trigeminal nerve (V_1) is called herpes zoster ophthalmicus (HZO). Ocular involvement occurs in about 70% of these patients.

■ Epidemiology
- Most patients are 60 to 90 years old, and the majority are healthy with no specific predisposing factors.
- Consider an immunocompromising condition, such as human immunodeficiency virus (HIV) infection or systemic malignancy, in affected patients younger than 40 years.

■ History
- Painful, vesicular rash with associated fever, headache, and malaise
- Possibly a red painful eye and/or blurry vision

■ Clinical Manifestations (see Table 7-1)
- Maculopapular rash in the CN V distribution, followed by vesicles, pustules, then crusting and scabbing; typically does not cross the midline (dermatomal).

- Vesicles on the eyelids may lead to secondary bacterial infection and/or eyelid inflammation.
  - Vesicals on tip of the nose (Hutchinson's sign) indicate involvement of the nasociliary branch of the ophthalmic division of CN V and may predict a higher risk of ocular involvement.
- Inflammation of almost any ocular tissue can occur and recur in HZO.
  - Conjunctivitis and/or pseudodendrites (may occur after resolution of skin lesions).
  - Punctate or dendritic keratitis: secondary to viral replication in corneal epithelium.
  - Round corneal infiltrates in stromal keratitis: chronic inflammation may lead to corneal vascularization/opacities.
  - Interstitial and disciform keratitis: not clinically distinguishable from that caused by HSV.
  - Corneal anesthesia in neurotrophic keratopathy.
  - Uveitis: iridocyclitis (Plate 1) and/or choroiditis.
  - Other ocular manifestations may include episcleritis, scleritis, retinitis, or optic neuritis.
  - Cranial nerve palsies, most commonly involving CN III, occur in about 30% of cases.

■ Risk Factors

- Age greater than 60 years
- Immunocompromise due to HIV, cancer, immunosuppressive therapy, or other debilitating factor

■ Differential Diagnosis

- HSV: skin lesions/vesicles often cross the midline and do not respect a dermatome. Has true dendritic keratitis, which stains brightly with fluorescein dye. Patients with HSV are typically younger.
- See discussion of differential diagnosis of HSV above.

■ Diagnostic Evaluation

- Ascertain if there is a history of immunocompromising disease or HIV. Ask about the duration of the rash and if it is associated with pain.
- Complete ophthalmic examination should focus on the cornea, signs of uveitis, and elevated IOP. Perform dilated fundus examination to rule out retinitis/optic neuritis.
- Patients younger than 40 years should be systemically evaluated for immunocompromising disease.

■ Treatment

- Famciclovir 500 mg PO three times per day or valacyclovir 1 g PO three times per day or acyclovir 800 mg PO five times per

day for 7 to 10 days. Ideally started within 72 hours of the onset of skin lesions.
  -Reduces viral shedding from vesicles, risk of systemic spread of virus, as well severity of ocular involvement/pain
- Intravenous acyclovir therapy is indicated in patients at risk for disseminated zoster due to immunosuppression.
- Topical antivirals are not effective.
- For skin lesions: warm compresses and topical antibiotic ointment (e.g., bacitracin or erythromycin 1 to 3 times per day) to prevent secondary infection.
- Keratitis and/or uveitis: topical steroid (e.g., prednisolone acetate 1%, one drop four times per day) and topical cyclo-plegic (e.g., cyclogel 1%, one drop 1 to 4 times per day) (may need steroid for 6 months or more).
- Neurotrophic keratopathy: lubrication, punctal occlusion, and possibly tarsorrhaphy.
- Postherpetic neuralgia: capsaicin 0.025% (e.g., Zostrix) cream to affected skin 2 to 4 times per day. Consider low-dose tri-cyclic antidepressant (e.g., amitriptyline 25 mg PO 3 times per day or anticonvulsant (e.g., phenytoin 100 mg PO 1 to 2 times per day).
- Corneal.

   Note: Patient should avoid contact with children, pregnant women, and adults without a history of chickenpox because varicella-zoster virus is contagious and can be spread by inhalation.

■ Follow-up
- Days to weeks, depending on severity
  -1 to 7 days if ocular involvement
  -1 to 4 weeks if no ocular involvement
  -3 to 6 months after resolution of episode

Contact Lens–Related Problems

Contact lens use predisposes patients to a variety of problems, including dry eye, giant papillary conjunctivitis (GPC), toxic conjunctivitis, corneal epithelial damage, infectious corneal infiltrates/ulcers, and corneal neovascularization.

■ History
- Dry/foreign body sensation, pain, photophobia, decreased vision
- Red eye, itching, discharge

■ Clinical Manifestations

- Conjunctival injection, corneal punctate epithelial staining.
- Corneal erosions, ulcers, infiltrates. Infiltrates/ulcers appear as white lesions that sometimes stain with fluorescein (Plate 3). Infiltrates/ulcers must always be ruled out with contact lens patients.
- Giant papillary conjunctivitis (GPC): itching, redness, and mucous discharge. Are often lens intolerant, especially if large papillae are present under the superior lid.
- Micropannus: neovascularization (usually superior) into peripheral cornea due to hypoxia and stress to the limbus; less than 2 mm is acceptable.

■ Risk Factors

- Overnight wear or prolonged use of lenses
- Poor lens cleaning/hygiene
- Use of home-made saline solution (increased rate of *Acanthamoeba* infection)

■ Differential Diagnosis

- Corneal infiltrate/ulcer (Plate 3): infectious or sterile infiltrates/ ulcers due to autoimmune disease
- Corneal foreign body: slit lamp examination can distinguish a foreign body from an infiltrate
- Blepharitis, conjunctivitis, dry eye syndrome

■ Diagnostic Evaluation

- History and slit lamp examination with and without contact lens
- Evert the upper eye lids to check for large papillae or the presence of foreign bodies
- Smears and cultures for suspicion or infectious ulcers/ infiltrates

   Note: All contact lens wearers with decreased vision, redness, pain, or discharge should immediately remove the contact lens and have an ophthalmic examination as soon as possible.

■ Treatment

- Discontinue or reduce use of contact lenses depending on condition.
- Topical mast cell stabilizer (e.g., olopatadine hydrochloride, one drop two times per day) or a topical NSAID (e.g., ketorolac tromethamine, one drop four times per day) for GPC.

- Broad-spectrum topical antibiotics (e.g., gatifloxacin, moxi-floxacin, or fortified antibiotics up to every hour) for infectious disease (e.g., corneal infiltrate/ulcers).
- Consider culture of suspicious infiltrates, especially if it is large, there is no epithelium, or it is in the visual axis of the cornea.

■ Follow-up

- Daily if corneal infection cannot be ruled out.
- Every 1 to 3 weeks if noninfectious entity.
- Closer follow-up if using topical steroids.
- Continue treatment until the process resolves.
- Discontinue contact lens wear until the process resolves.

8

Glaucoma

Thomas E. Bournias, MD

GLAUCOMA

Glaucoma refers to a group of diseases that have in common a characteristic optic neuropathy manifested by loss of retinal ganglion cells. There may or may not be associated visual field loss (early glaucoma is defined as a glaucomatous-appearing optic nerve without associated visual field changes). Elevated intraocular pressure (IOP) may or may not be present. Therefore, elevated IOP is considered a risk factor and is not necessarily causative. Other risk factors include advanced age, racial background (increased risk in blacks), glaucoma in the opposite eye, a larger cup/disc ratio, and a positive family history. Normally, IOP falls in the range of 10 to 21 mm Hg. IOP can fluctuate ±6 mm Hg in normal individuals and even more in glaucoma patients. About 60% to 70% of glaucomas are associated with elevated IOP leaving another 30% to 40% never having had elevated IOP (normal-tension glaucoma). A significant number of people have elevated IOP (22 mm Hg or higher) but do not develop glaucoma.

Left untreated, for most patients, it is an asymptomatic disease with slow progressive loss of peripheral vision (which may go unnoticed for years) until finally resulting in "tunnel vision" and eventual blindness. It is important to carefully monitor the optic nerve and visual field for progressive changes consistent with glaucoma.

Characteristic changes of the optic nerve indicating the presence or progression of glaucoma include generalized enlargement of the cup/disc ratio, loss of neuroretinal rim tissue and nerve fiber layer, notching of the optic nerve, disc hemorrhage, and baring of the circumlinear vessel (loss of rim tissue resulting in a vessel that was previously in the neuroretinal rim now isolated within the cup). Most normal nerves have a characteristic neuroretinal rim (Figure 8-1). Because there is a round cup located in a vertically elongated oval optic disc, the width of the neural rim tissue varies by quadrant. In the normal eye, the neural rim is thickest in the Inferior quadrant, followed in descending order by the Superior, Nasal, and Temporal (ISN'T rule). A nerve with a larger cup/disc ratio whose neuroretinal rim does not follow this rule is

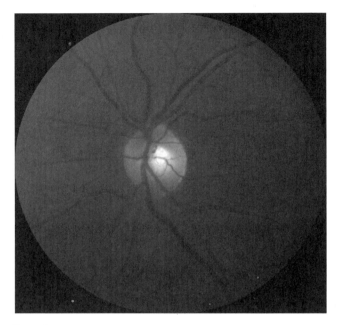

Figure 8-1 • Normal left nerve. Note a small cup/disc ratio of about 0.3. The neuroretina rim follows the "ISN'T" rule I > S > N > T.

suspicious for glaucomatous change (Figure 8-2). Glaucomatous optic nerves generally have a greater cup/disc ratio (e.g., 0.5) than normal optic nerves (e.g., 0.3).

Typical visual field findings include generalized suppression, nasal step, Seidel's scotoma, arcuate defect and later paracentral defects, split fixation, and small islands of vision (in advanced glaucoma) (Figure 8-3).

Primary glaucoma is classified as open angle and narrow angle. Aqueous humor is produced in the ciliary body and flows through the pupil to fill the anterior chamber (AC) and eventually drain through the trabecular meshwork (TM) and uveoscleral outflow pathways (Figures 8-4 and 8-5). In open-angle glaucoma, IOP is elevated as a result of resistance in the TM. In narrow-angle glaucoma (or angle-closure glaucoma), the TM is obstructed such as in pupillary block. Here aqueous builds in the posterior chamber resulting in anterior bowing of the iris and subsequent obstruction of the angle. Other conditions (e.g., rubeosis iridis) can block the TM resulting in elevated IOP.

Treatment is recommended if the patient has elevated IOP without glaucoma (but is at high risk), has glaucoma and demonstrates

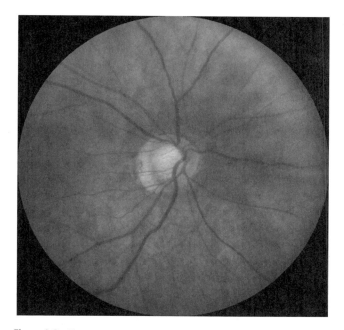

Figure 8-2 • Glaucomatous right nerve.

progression, or has significant damage that may alter his or her function or quality of life or result in blindness. IOP reduction is the treatment for all glaucomas (including normal-tension glaucoma) if attempting to halt or slow progressive changes in the optic nerve/visual field.

Medications are usually chosen first (Table 8-1) with topical prostaglandin analogs-hypotensive lipids generally being the most potent and safest systemically. Laser trabeculoplasty may be performed before or after the initiation of medication (see p. 173) and incisional surgery is generally reserved for patients who progress despite maximally tolerated medical therapy, are intolerant to medical therapy, or are noncompliant with or cannot afford medication. (See Chapter 12 for glaucoma procedures.)

Primary Open-Angle Glaucoma

In primary open-angle glaucoma (POAG), there are glaucomatous optic nerve changes with/without associated visual field changes usually in the setting of IOP being 22 mm Hg or higher. POAG accounts for 60% to 70% of open-angle glaucomas.

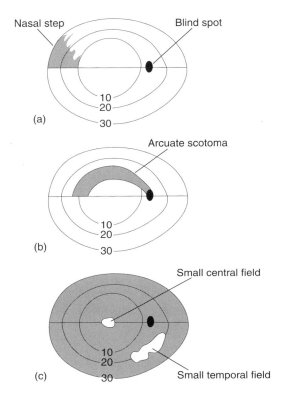

Figure 8-3 • Visual field loss in glaucoma often demonstrates a characteristic pattern. For example, loss of fibers in the inferior pole of the optic nerve may results in (a) a superior nasal step. With progression the nasal step may develop into to (b) an arcuate scotoma and later to a (c) a small central island of vision (tunnel vision). Sometimes there may be sparing of a small temporal island of vision.

■ History

- Usually asymptomatic initially.
- Decreased peripheral vision or central vision later in disease.
- Tunnel vision only late in the disease when both visual fields are severely damaged.
- Central fixation is typically preserved until very late in the disease.

■ Clinical Manifestations

- Normal anterior ocular examination.
- IOP usually 22 mm Hg or higher.
- Large diurnal (different IOP readings throughout the day) fluctuations in IOP (IOP may fluctuate ± 6 mm Hg or more,

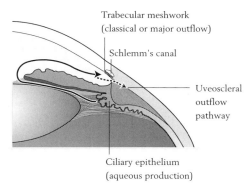

Figure 8-4 • Route of aqueous production in the ciliary body to drainage in the trabecular meshwork and uveoscleral outflow.

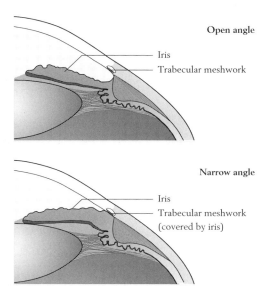

Figure 8-5 • Classification of primary glaucoma. There is no iris obstruction to the trabecular meshwork in open-angle glaucoma. In narrow-angle glaucoma, the iris physically obstructs the trabecular meshwork (e.g., pupillary block in angle closure or rubeosis irides in neovascular glaucoma).

■ TABLE 8-1 Glaucoma Medications

Medication	Classification	Mechanism of Action
Topical		
Pilocarpine 1–6%	Cholinergic	Outflow facility
Carbachol	Cholinergic	Outflow facility
Dipivefrin (e.g., Propine)	Nonselective adrenergic	Outflow facility
Apraclonidine (e.g., Iopidine)	Selective adrenergic	Aqueous suppressant
Brimonidine (e.g., Alphagan-P)	Selective adrenergic	Aqueous suppressant/ uveoscleral outflow
Timolol (e.g., Timoptic XE)	Beta blocker	Aqueous suppressant
Dorzolamide (Trusoptl) or Brinzolamide (Azopt)	Carbonic anhydrase inhibitor	Aqueous suppressant
Latanoprost (Xalatan), travoprost (Travatan)	Hypotensive lipid (prostaglandin)	Uveoscleral outflow
Bimatoprost (Lumigan)	Hypotensive lipid (prostamide)	Outflow facility/ uveoscleral outflow
Unoprostone isopropyl (Rescula)	Hypotensive lipid (Decosanoid)	Outflow facility
Oral		
Acetazolamide (e.g., Diamox)	Carbonic anhydrase inhibitor	Aqueous suppressant
Isosorbide	Hyperosmotic	Osmotic

See Appendix C for indications, side effects, and other drug information.

therefore some readings may be in the normal range at various times of day).
- Open angle on gonioscopy without peripheral anterior synechia (PAS). PAS are areas of scarring in the drainage angle resulting from narrow angles, inflammation, or other processes. These scars obstruct the TM.
- Optic nerve changes as discussed above.
- Visual field defects as discussed above.

Note: Diurnal refers to the different IOP readings at different times of the day. It is recommended that all patients have their diurnal curve checked so that fluctuations of their IOP can be recorded.

■ Risk Factors
- Family history of glaucoma or blindness
- Glaucoma in the contralateral eye
- Black race
- Diabetes, hypertension (vascular disease)
- Older age
- Larger cup/disc ratio (e.g., ≥0.5)

■ Differential Diagnosis

- Ocular hypertension: IOP is elevated but the optic nerve and visual field are normal.
- Normal-tension glaucoma: same findings in POAG but IOP is consistently less than 22 mm Hg.
- Physiologic optic nerve cupping: cup/disc ratio is enlarged but IOP is normal. Large cup/disc ratios are seen in myopic discs and larger optic nerves (about 2.0 mm; smaller optic nerves are about 1.0 mm in diameter). This condition has no notching of the optic nerve rim and does not change over time. The optic nerve appearance follows the "ISN'T" rule (see above). Visual fields are normal.
- Secondary open-angle glaucoma: other types of open-angle glaucoma such as pigmentary, exfoliative, angle recession, steroid induced, and so forth.
- Chronic angle-closure glaucoma: same findings in POAG except AC angle on gonioscopy demonstrates narrow angle with PAS. Does not develop acute, sudden rise in IOP with pain as in acute angle-closure glaucoma.
- Optic atrophy: IOP is usually normal; usually more pallor of the optic nerve than cupping. Visual field loss more typical of atrophy or compressive tumor than glaucoma. Visual field defects usually worse than expected, given the amount of optic nerve cupping. Altitudinal visual field defects are more common for anterior ischemic optic neuropathies. Altitudinal defects respecting the vertical midline are more typical of intracranial lesions in the visual pathways. Optic atrophy is often seen in ischemic optic neuropathy, syphilis, chiasmal tumor, and so forth.
- Previous optic nerve damage: damage occurred previously from elevated IOP secondary to a modality that has been eliminated (e.g., steroid, uveitis, trauma).
- Congenital optic nerve defects: e.g., myopic discs, optic nerve pits, colobomas. In these conditions, IOP is usually normal. If a visual field defect exists, it does not progress.
- Optic nerve drusen: often visible clinically and optic nerves usually are not cupped. May have visual field defects. Calcification of the optic disc may be seen by B-scan ultrasound or computed tomography (CT).

■ Diagnostic Evaluation

- Determine if there are risk factors present, such as family history, cardiovascular disease, previously elevated IOP, or steroid use.
- Check IOP and diurnal curve (multiple IOP measurements at different times of the day).
- Examination: gonioscopy to verify that the angle is open without PAS. Dilated fundus examination to evaluate the optic nerve and nerve fiber layer.

- Visual field testing to look for nasal, paracentral, or arcuate defects.
- Stereo disc photos (SDPs) to document the appearance of the optic nerve and nerve fiber layer.
- In addition to SDPs, consider computerized imaging techniques, such as Heidelberg retinal tomography (HRT), ocular coherence tomography (OCT), and GDx.

Note: Some clinicians perform pachymetry of the central cornea in glaucoma patients. Studies have shown that IOP readings from Goldmann applanation tonometers may be altered by the corneal thickness (see Tonometry in Chapter 2). The benefit of this has not been established in glaucoma patients as it has in ocular hypertensives (without glaucoma).

■ Treatment

Lower the IOP (the only proven treatment): The usual goal is an initial 20% to 40% reduction in IOP from baseline depending on the severity of the glaucoma. The type and aggressiveness of treatment are determined by the baseline IOP, the amount of damage already present, the rate of progression, and the anticipated life expectancy of the patient.

- Topical medications as listed in Table 8-1.
    - Hypotensive lipids are often used first because they are generally the most effective.
    - Beta-blockers, alpha-agonists, and carbonic anhydrase inhibitors are often added (if necessary) in various combinations.
- Oral carbonic anhydrase inhibitors (e.g., acetazolamide 250 mg PO four times per day) are associated with more systemic side effects.
- Laser trabeculoplasty (may be used before or after treatment with topical medication):
    - Argon laser trabeculoplasty: thermal treatment to TM
    - Selective laser trabeculoplasty: nonthermal treatment to TM. This form of trabeculoplasty may be repeatable.
- Incisional surgery is usually considered if medical and laser therapy are not adequate (see Chapter 12).
    - Trabeculectomy
    - Aqueous shunt
- Cyclodestructive (ciliary ablation) procedures are considered if incisional surgery is ineffective, likely to fail, or the eye is blind and painful.
    - Cyclocryotherapy (freezing)
    - Transscleral cyclophotocoagulation (diode laser)
- Consider systemic workup if the optic nerves and/or visual fields look more consistent with neurologic signs/symptoms (especially in the presence of normal IOP).

■ Follow-up

- Acutely, with very high IOP (more than 35 mm Hg) plus or minus moderate to advanced glaucomatous cupping: 1 to 7 days.
- IOP not adequately controlled or to evaluate initiation or change in therapy: 1 to 6 weeks.
- Routine follow-up for controlled IOP: 3 to 6 months.
- Perform serial visual fields and SDPs (or HRT, OCT, GDx).
  - Visual fields are performed one to four times per year, depending on the severity of the glaucomatous damage.
  - SDPs (or HRT, OCT, GDx) are generally performed yearly.

Ocular Hypertension

Elevated IOP (higher than 22 mm Hg) without glaucomatous optic nerve or visual field changes. Ten percent of all untreated ocular hypertensive patients (IOP from 24–32 mm Hg) will develop a glaucomatous optic nerve or visual field in 5 years.

■ History

- Asymptomatic
- May develop glaucoma with optic nerve changes and/or visual field loss

■ Clinical Manifestations

- Normal external ocular examination
- IOP usually greater than 22 mm Hg
- Open angle by gonioscopy without PAS
- Healthy optic nerve and nerve fiber layer (optic nerve appearance usually follows "ISN'T" rule)
- Normal visual field testing

■ Risk Factors

- See Primary Open-Angle Glaucoma.
- Thinner central corneal thickness (CCT)
  - Patients with a CCT less than 555 µm by contact ultrasound pachymetry have an overall threefold increased risk than a patient with a CCT greater than 588 µm.
- Greater cup/disc ratio
- Older age

■ Differential Diagnosis

- POAG: glaucoma present but with minimal optic nerve or visual field changes.

- Narrow angle: no glaucoma present but narrow angle present on gonioscopy with/without PAS. IOP is often intermittantly elevated.
- Pseudoexfoliation (PXE) without glaucoma: essentially the eye appears normal except small white flecks may be seen on the pupillary border, lens, or corneal endothelium. Gonioscopic examination usually reveals an open angle with increased pigmentation, often with a Sampaolesi's line (pigment anterior to Schwalbe's line).
- Pigment dispersion without glaucoma: no glaucoma present but may see pigment on the corneal endothelium (Krukenberg's spindle). Iris may demonstrate midperipheral transillumination defects. Gonioscopic examination usually reveals an open angle with increased pigmentation, often with a Sampaolesi's line.
- Current or recent use of intravenous, oral, topical drops, ointment, or inhaled steroids: IOP may be greatly increased in about 15% of individuals using any type of steroid, usually for 6 or more weeks (but may occur with shorter duration of use).

■ Diagnostic Evaluation

- See Primary Open-Angle Glaucoma.
- Pachymetric testing to determine CCT.
- Baseline SDPs and visual field (VF) testing (if VF has a defect that does not appear consistent with the optic nerve, repeat it as there is a learning curve for taking visual fields).
- Consider other imaging modalities (e.g., HRT, OCT, GDx) of the optic nerve.

Note: A recent study showed that measuring CCT in ocular hypertensive patients (without glaucoma) may help predict which patients with ocular hypertension may develop glaucomatous optic nerve or visual field changes and need subsequent treatment. Higher risk patients have a CCT less than 555 μm and lower risk patients have a CCT greater than 588 μm. This benefit of pachymetry in true glaucoma patients has not been established.

■ Treatment

- Observation in lower to moderate-risk individuals.
- Consider treatment in higher risk individuals.
  - Thinner CCT: less than 555 μm
  - Older patients
  - Worse pattern standard deviation on visual field
  - Larger cup/disc ratio (e.g., greater than 0.5)
  - Higher baseline IOP

- Consider treatment in older persons with vascular disease to prevent a possible central retinal vein occlusion (CRVO).
- If treatment is initiated, the goal is about a 20% reduction in IOP from baseline with topical medications and/or laser trabeculoplasty (ALT or SLT).

▣ Follow-up
- 3 to 12 months initially
- 6 to 12 months if stable after a few years
- Annual optic nerve evaluation and visual field testing

Normal-Pressure Glaucoma

Glaucoma with IOP consistently less than 22 mm Hg

▣ Epidemiology
- Usually individuals older than 50 years
- Accounts for about 30% to 40% of open-angle glaucomas
- More common in Japanese

▣ History
- Usually asymptomatic
- Glaucomatous optic nerve cupping and/or visual field loss despite IOPs consistently less than 22 mm Hg

▣ Clinical Manifestations
- See Primary Open-Angle Glaucoma.
- IOP always less than 22 mm Hg.
- Visual field defects: usually nasal or paracentral. Often arcuate, extending from the blind spot to the nasal periphery.

▣ Risk Factors
- See Primary Open-Angle Glaucoma.
- Vasospastic disorders (e.g., Raynaud's phenomenon, migraines).

▣ Differential Diagnosis
- POAG: IOP may be less than 22 mm Hg at different times of day.
- Angle-closure glaucoma: patients often with intermittent episodes of blurred vision, halos, pain, and redness. Gonioscopic examination reveals narrow angles, often with PAS.
- Previous ischemia to optic nerve: e.g., a previous ischemic optic neuropathy or hypotensive event. The patient may have experienced sudden visual loss. The optic nerve usually demonstrates more pallor than cupping. Optic nerve changes usually do not progress, but the contralateral eye may become

involved. Visual field defects may appear glaucomatous or altitudinal.

- Previous elevated IOP producing glaucomatous damage: history of trauma, uveitis, steroid use, glaucomatocyclitic crisis.
- Syphilis: slit lamp examination may demonstrate old corneal blood vessels devoid of blood (ghost vessels) or evidence of old iritis (posterior or anterior synechia or pigment on the lens). Dilated fundus examination may demonstrate salt-and-pepper appearance of retina. Optic nerves may appear cupped/pale. Will have a positive FTA-ABS.
- Compressive optic neuropathy: possibly from a tumor or aneurysm. Pallor of the optic nerve usually more prominent than cupping. Visual field defects usually do not look glaucomatous and often respect the vertical meridian (unlike glaucoma).
- Hematologic disease: the optic nerve may appear cupped in anemia.

■ Diagnostic Evaluation

See Primary Open-Angle Glaucoma.

■ Treatment

- Observation: If the diagnosis is in question, another explanation for the glaucomatous change exists, the glaucoma is progressing slowly without significant visual field loss, or the patient is older with minimal field loss.
- Treatment may be indicated for:
  - Advanced optic nerve cupping
  - Visual field defect encroaching on central vision
  - Cupping/field loss unexplained by another disease
  - Younger patient with significant field loss
  - Rapid progression of cupping/visual field loss
  - Appearance of a disc hemorrhage.
- Goal of initial treatment is about a 30% reduction in IOP.
- Laser trabeculoplasty tends to have little efficacy.
- Medicine and incisional surgery are generally more effective.

■ Follow-up

- 3 to 6 months

Steroid Responder Glaucoma

IOP may increase within 2 to 6 weeks of initiating steroid therapy including inhaled, repository, ointment, topical, oral, or intravenous forms. The elevated IOP is due to resistance at the TM. Severe damage may occur with prolonged use.

■ **Epidemiology**

- 15% of population at risk for significant IOP elevation with steroid use.
- Patients with POAG or associated risk factors have a higher risk of developing a steroid response.

■ **History**

- Elevated IOP within a few weeks (sometimes within days to months) of initiating steroid therapy.
- Glaucomatous optic neuropathy and/or visual field loss may occur during this time.
- IOP often returns to normal within days to weeks of discontinuing therapy, but may remain elevated for months.

■ **Clinical Manifestations**

- Elevated IOP (often more than 30 mm Hg).
- Normal angle by gonioscopy.
- Evidence of open-angle glaucoma may develop: optic nerve cupping and/or visual field loss.

■ **Differential Diagnosis**

- See Primary Open-Angle Glaucoma.
- Inflammatory open-angle glaucoma: elevated IOP may be secondary to the inflammation or the steroid treatment.

■ **Diagnostic Evaluation**

- Inquire about any history of steroid use and duration.
- Slit lamp examination: determine if there is inflammation in the AC or evidence of iris neovascularization. Measure the IOP.
- Gonioscopic examination to determine if angle neovascularization is present.
- Dilated fundus examination to evaluate the optic nerve for glaucomatous change.
- Formal visual field testing and SDPs (or HRT, OCT, GDx).

■ **Treatment**

- Taper steroid use as safely and rapidly as possible.
- Reduce the dose or concentration of the steroid.
- Try a steroid with a lower incidence of IOP elevation (e.g., loteprednol etabonate 0.5% instead of prednisolone acetate 1%).
- Switch to a topical nonsteroidal formula (e.g., ketorolac tromethamine, diclofenac sodium) if anti-inflammatory medication required.

- Initiate antiglaucoma therapy if IOP remains dangerously high despite the use of above measures or if glaucomatous optic nerve or visual field changes occur.
- To determine if IOP elevation is secondary to the steroid or inflammation, consider increasing the steroid therapy. If IOP elevation remains, despite a reduction in inflammation, the raised IOP is more to likely to be steroid induced.

Note: Always demonstrate caution when injecting periocular depot steroids. If the patient is a steroid responder, the depot may have to be surgically excised. An individual on any chronic steroid (greater than two weeks) should have careful ophthalmic follow-up.

■ Follow-up
- Daily if IOP elevated (more than 35 mm Hg) and uncontrolled.
- Discontinue any unnecessary steroids.
- Every 3 to 6 months when stable.

Pigment Dispersion Syndrome

In pigment dispersion syndrome (PDS), a pathologic increase in TM pigment results in elevated IOP. It is thought that the iris assumes a concave position, allowing pigment on the posterior iris to rub against the zonules and disperse into the aqueous to subsequently block the TM.

■ Epidemiology
- More common in men aged 20 to 55 years
- More common in myopic individuals; usually bilateral

■ History
- Often asymptomatic
- Occasionally blurred vision, halos around lights or eye pain after pupillary dilation or exercise

■ Clinical Manifestations
- Spokelike transillumination defects (Plate 13) in the midperipheral iris
- Vertical pigmented band on corneal endothelium (Krukenberg's spindle)
- Pigment deposition on equatorial lens surface (line of Zentmyer)
- Gonioscopy: open angles with dense pigmentation of TM and possible Sampaolesi's line
- IOP spikes (pigmented cells may be seen in AC as well as corneal edema during IOP spikes)
- Glaucoma (optic nerve cupping with visual field loss)

■ **Differential Diagnosis**

- Pseudoexfoliative (PXE) glaucoma: may have unilaterally elevated IOP. Slit lamp examination reveals white flaky material on the corneal endothelium, pupillary border, or lens. Transillumination defects tend to be closer to papillary border. Gonioscopy similar to PDS.
- Inflammatory open-angle glaucoma: white blood cells in AC without iris transillumination defects. Gonioscopic examination may reveal PAS.
- Iris melanoma: Gonioscopic examination reveals increased pigment in the angle with areas of darkened iris.

■ **Diagnostic Evaluation**

- Ascertain if there is a history of any previous episodes of halos or loss of vision, especially with exercise.
- Slit lamp examination: check for Krukenberg's spindle on endothelium or iris transillumination defects by obtaining a red reflex by shining a small slit beam directly into the pupil. Transillumination defects may now be evident in the midperipheral iris.
- Measure IOP.
- Perform gonioscopy to verify angle is open and increased pigmentation of the TM (and possible Sampaolesi's line).
- Dilated funduscopic examination: evaluate the optic nerve and examine peripheral retina for holes, or breaks, or lattice (thin areas of peripheral retina) as these patients tend to be myopic with an increased risk of these findings.
- Baseline SDPs (or HRT, OCT, GDx).

■ **Treatment**

- As in open-angle glaucoma above. Observation if IOP is not too high and the optic nerve is healthy. Amount of IOP reduction is based on the level of glaucomatous damage and level of risk.
- Topical antiglaucoma medications usually used first (e.g., hypotensive lipids, beta blockers, alpha agonists).
- Miotics (e.g., pilocarpine) have theoretical advantages because they reduce contact of the iris with the lens zonules and thereby decrease release of pigment granules into the AC. However, miotics are not practical because they can increase myopia in younger patients. Use miotics in myopic individuals with caution as they may cause retinal tears or detachments.
- Argon or selective laser trabeculoplasty may be employed as initial therapy because pigment dispersion responds very well to laser trabeculoplasty (more than 90% of patients).
- Laser peripheral iridectomy has been advocated for theoretical reasons because it can eliminate the reverse papillary block and

decrease iridozonular contact with resultant pigment dispersion. Only individuals with active pigment dispersion and a
concave iris configuration on gonioscopy may benefit from this
procedure (less than 10% of patients with PDS).
- Trabeculectomy is indicated when medical or laser therapy has
failed in glaucomatous eyes.

■ **Follow-up**
- Elevated IOP without glaucoma: every 6 to 12 months with a
visual field annually
- With glaucomatous damage: every 3 to 6 months with a visual
field every 6 to 12 months

Pseudoexfoliative Glaucoma (Exfoliative Glaucoma)

Pseudoexfoliative glaucoma is a condition in which a white, flaky,
fibrillar material is found on structures in the anterior segment of
the eye including the corneal endothelium, iris, lens, ciliary
epithelium, and angle structures. This material resembles
amyloid, and its presence gives an increased risk of developing
elevated IOP with a resultant sixfold increased risk of developing
glaucoma. The cause of the elevated IOP is unknown.

■ **Epidemiology**
- Usually unilateral (may be bilateral with varying degrees of
asymmetry).
- More common in people of Scandinavian, northern European,
and Russian descent.
- Incidence increases with age.

■ **History**
- Usually asymptomatic

■ **Clinical Manifestations**
- Slit lamp examination reveals white flaky material on the
pupillary border and anterior lens capsule. Distinct pattern on
lens often seen upon dilation: central zone of exfoliation material, middle clear zone, a peripheral cloudy zone (Figure 8-6).
Transillumination defects may be seen along the pupillary
border.
- IOP may be normal to elevated (may be greater than 60 mm
Hg).
- Gonioscopic examination demonstrates increased pigment deposition on the TM and anterior to Schwalbe's line (Sampaolesi's
line).

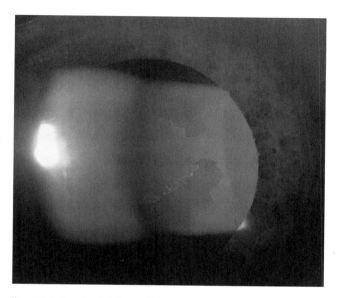

Figure 8-6 • Pseudoexfoliation syndrome may reveal flaky fibrillar material on the lens, pupil border, corneal endothelium, and ciliary body. Here a typical "target" appearance on the lens is seen. There are three distinct zones: (1) a translucent, central disc; (2) a clear zone corresponding to the moving iris; and (3) a peripheral granular zone.

- Dilated fundus examination may reveal optic nerve cupping.
- Visual field testing may demonstrate glaucomatous changes.

■ Differential Diagnosis

- Pigmentary glaucoma: Midperipheral transillumination defects of the iris in contrast to along pupillary border as seen in pseudoexfoliation. Vertical pigmented band may be seen on corneal endothelium (Krukenberg's spindle). Gonioscopic features similar to those of pseudoexfoliation.
- Capsular delamination (true exfoliation): a thin membrane of the anterior lens capsule peels off secondary to intense heat (e.g., glass blower), trauma, or uveitis.
- Primary amyloidosis: similar findings of flaky white material with possible increased IOP.

■ Diagnostic Evaluation

- Ascertain if there is a history of trauma or occupational exposure to heat.

- Slit lamp examination: look for transillumination defects along pupillary border and white flaky material on corneal endothelium, pupillary border, and lens.
- Measure IOP and perform gonioscopic examination looking for increased pigmentation.
- Funduscopic evaluation of the optic nerve for glaucomatous change.
- Baseline SDPs and visual fields.

■ Treatment

- Same for POAG.
- Laser trabeculoplasty (argon or selective) is more effective with a higher initial success rate (more than 90%) than POAG (about 80% successful at one year).
- Trabeculectomy when medical or laser therapy is not effective.

■ Follow-up

- Every 1 to 4 months as determined by severity of the glaucoma.
- Exfoliation syndrome without glaucoma examined every 6 to 12 months because of increased risk of developing glaucoma. IOP tends to increase as the patient gets older.

Acute Angle-Closure Glaucoma

Acute rise in IOP secondary to obstruction of the TM by the iris. Aqueous cannot pass between the iris and lens. A buildup of aqueous collects behind the iris resulting in anterior bowing of the iris and resultant narrowing of the anterior chamber angle and blockage of the TM.

■ Epidemiology

- Accounts for less than 1% of glaucoma in whites
- More common in Asians, Eskimos, and hyperopes (shorter axial length)

■ History

- Severe eye pain with frontal headache
- Blurred vision with colored halos around lights
- Nausea and vomiting

■ Clinical Manifestations

- External examination demonstrates conjunctival injection (with possible ciliary flush) and a fixed, middilated pupil.
- Slit lamp examination reveals microcystic corneal edema and a shallow anterior chamber.

- The anterior chamber angle is closed on gonioscopic examination in the involved eye. The angle is often narrow in the contralateral eye.
- IOP is usually elevated above 35 mm Hg.
- Visual loss and glaucomatous optic neuropathy may occur in hours.

■ Risk Factors

- History of angle closure in opposite eye
- Hyperopia with a narrow angle
- May be precipitated by topical mydriatics in an eye with a narrow angle
- Rarely precipitated by miotics or systemic anticholinergics (e.g., antihistamines or cold medications)

■ Differential Diagnosis

These entities often have an acute rise in IOP in one eye. However, gonioscopic examination reveals the angle to be open.

- Glaucomatocyclitic crisis (Posner-Schlossman syndrome): intermittent IOP spikes in one eye. Eye is generally not red and not painful. Slit lamp examination reveals mild anterior chamber cell and flare with or without keratic precipitates.
- Inflammatory open-angle glaucoma: anterior uveitis in one eye with acute elevation in intraocular pressure. Pupil may be miotic and slit lamp examination reveals cell and flare in the anterior chamber and possibly keratic precipitates on the posterior surface of the corneal endothelium. Gonioscopic examination may sometimes reveal PAS, however.
- Traumatic (hemolytic) glaucoma: patient with recent history of blunt trauma to the eye. Slit lamp examination may reveal red blood cells in the anterior chamber.
- Pigmentary glaucoma: after exercise or pupillary dilation, pigmentary cells may be seen floating in the anterior chamber on slit lamp examination.

■ Diagnostic Evaluation

- Ascertain if there have been episodes of eye pain, blurred vision, halos, nausea, or vomiting. Determine if there is any recent medication use.
- Perform slit lamp examination to determine if the anterior chamber is shallow or if there is cell and flare. Look for keratic precipitates, iris neovascularization, posterior synechiae, or a swollen lens.
- Record IOP.
- Perform gonioscopic examination on both eyes as the contralateral eye may have a narrow angle.

- May need to defer dilated fundus examination; but when performed, examine optic nerve for degree of damage and for evidence of a central retinal vein occlusion.

■ Treatment

- Aggressive IOP reduction with topical medications.
- Topical steroids (e.g., prednisolone acetate 1%) up to every hour.
- If attack is of recent onset and minimal corneal edema is present, corneal compression with a gonioprism may be attempted. This may help open the angle and reduce the IOP.
- If IOP is still elevated despite topical medications, consider acetazolamide orally (e.g., 250–500 mg in one dose) or intravenously (e.g., 250–500 mg in one injection).
- If IOP is still elevated, consider an osmotic agent (e.g., isosorbide 50–100 mg PO or mannitol 1–2 g/kg IV over 45 minutes).
- If gonioscopic examination reveals a closed angle, definitive treatment is laser peripheral iridectomy (LPI) with argon or Nd:YAG (neodymium:yttrium-aluminium-garnet) laser.
- The contralateral eye usually receives an LPI soon after or first if the cornea is too swollen to allow visualization for a PI on the involved eye.
- Surgical iridectomy if a laser PI is not possible.
- Consider laser gonioplasty or filtration surgery (trabeculectomy) if IOP remains high despite laser PI and institution of maximal medical therapy.
- In cases of phacomorphic glaucoma (a large lens pushing the lens-iris diaphragm forward, resulting in angle closure), the lens should urgently be removed.

Note: *Acute angle-closure glaucoma is an urgent emergency.* **Acute IOP greater than 35 mm Hg must be managed aggressively as permanent visual loss may ensue in hours. The patient's cardiovascular status and electrolyte balance should be considered when employing beta blockers, carbonic anhydrase inhibitors, and osmotic agents.**

■ Follow-up

- Daily until definitive treatment performed and IOP controlled.
- After definitive treatment performed, patient is seen in weeks to months initially.
- When stable, patients may be seen every 3 to 6 months.
- Baseline SDPs and visual fields are obtained.

9

Uveitis

Thomas E. Bournias, MD, Charlie Abraham, MD, and
Preeya Kshettry

Uveitis

The iris, choroid, and ciliary body form the uveal tract. Inflammation of one or more of the three components of the uveal tract is called uveitis. Uveitis can be classified according to the affected structure. Inflammation of the iris is termed anterior uveitis (iritis or iridocyclitis). Intermediate uveitis (cyclitis) encompasses inflammation in the region of the vitreous base and the inferior pars plana (posterior ciliary body). Finally, posterior uveitis involves inflammation of the posterior segment including the choroid, retina, and vitreous. Concurrent anterior and posterior uveitis is termed panuveitis. Uveitis may occur in association with inflammation of the overlying retina (retinitis) or of the optic nerve (optic neuritis).

■ Etiology

- Idiopathic: accounts for about one half of all cases of uveitis
- Infection: one of the following:
  - Bacteria
    - Tuberculosis (TB): chest x-ray and purified protein derivative (PPD) test help confirm the diagnosis. TB is more likely to cause posterior uveitis.
    - Syphilis: usually associated with maculopapular rash on the palms and soles. Positive VDRL or RPR and positive FTA-ABS are usually present. Syphilis is more likely to cause chorioretinitis and vitritis.
    - Lyme disease.
    - Reiter's syndrome: associated with a triad of urethritis, polyarthritis, and mucosal inflammation (such as conjunctivitis). It is often associated with iritis (40%). May also occur after bacterial infection such as chlamydia.
  - Viruses
    - Herpes simplex/varicella-zoster: usually associated with dendritic keratitis and skin vesicles. Caution for acute retinal necrosis.
    - Cytomegalovirus: develop retinitis with possible vitritis.

-Fungi
  -Candidiasis: usually presents with multifocal retinal lesions that may spread to the vitreous
  -Coccidioidomycosis
  -Aspergillosis
-Parasites
  -Toxoplasmosis: although the central nervous system is most often affected, the eye is a common organ targeted by toxoplasmosis. The retina and the choroid are most commonly affected. There is often vitritis.
  -Histoplasmosis: develops a triad of small, atrophic, punched-out chorioretinal scars in the midperiphery and posterior pole; peripapillary chorioretinal scarring; and choroidal neovascularization. There is no vitreous inflammation.
- Systemic inflammatory disease: usually immunologic tests are required to confirm the diagnosis.
  -Sarcoidosis: a granulomatous disease that affects many organs, especially the lungs, skin, and eyes. Ocular involvement in sarcoidosis generally occurs early in the disease course. (See Chapter 11, Sarcoidosis, pp. 163–165)
  -Ankylosing spondylitis: complain of stiffness at rest and sore back upon waking
  -Behçet's disease: generalize occlusive vasculitis of unknown cause associated with the classic triad of acute hypopyon iritis, aphthous stomatitis (cankerlike mouth ulcers), and genital ulceration. It is common in the Near East and Japan.
  -Others include: inflammatory bowel disease (Crohn's disease or ulcerative colitis), psoriatic arthritis, juvenile rheumatoid arthritis (JRA).
- Other
  -Postoperatively: can occur after any intraocular surgery such as cataract or glaucoma and pars plana vitrectomy. With improved surgical techniques, antibiotics, and other preoperative prophylactic medications, the incidence of postoperative uveitis has significantly decreased.
  -Immunocompromised patients (e.g., people with acquired immunodeficiency syndrome or on chemotherapy) have a higher risk of viral (e.g., cytomegalovirus), fungal (e.g., *Candida*), and endogenous bacterial uveitis.
  -Exposure to toxins, intraocular foreign bodies or medications (e.g., Sulfonamides, Rifabutin).

■ Epidemiology

- Anterior uveitis accounts for 75% of all cases of uveitis.
- Fifty percent of all cases of uveitis are associated with a systemic disease.

Note: As anterior uveitis accounts for the majority of all cases of uveitis, the remainder of this chapter will focus primarily on the workup and management of anterior uveitis.

■ History

- Acute onset of pain
- Light sensitivity (photophobia), tearing
- Blurry vision
- Redness, no purulent discharge is seen
- Floaters (in posterior uveitis) secondary to white blood cells and opacities in the vitreous

■ Clinical Manifestations

- Visual acuity may be slightly decreased.
- IOP is usually decreased and may occasionally be elevated.
- Conjunctival injection, especially bulbar conjunctiva (often a characteristic "ciliary flush" around the limbus).
- Keratic precipitates (KPs) may be present (white blood cells accumulated on the corneal endothelium).
- Corneal edema may be present.
- White blood cells (WBCs) and/or flare (protein) in the anterior chamber (AC) (Plate 1); WBCs may layer in the AC (hypopyon).
- Signs of iris inflammation may be present, such as posterior synechia (iris adhesion to the anterior lens capsule).
- Posterior subcapsular cataract formation with chronic inflammation (Plate 14).
- Signs of posterior uveitis include: WBCs in the vitreous (vitritis), disc swelling, retinal/choroidal infiltrates and retinal hemorrhages/exudates.

■ Differential Diagnosis

Entities associated with an AC reaction:

- Rhegmatogenous retinal detachment: pigmented cells may be seen in the AC or vitreous (Plate 2) in the presence of an elevated retina with a break.
- Pigment dispersion syndrome: often associated with pigmented cells in the AC.
- Intraocular foreign body: may stimulate an inflammatory reaction in the AC or vitreous.
- Endophthalmitis: intraocular inflammation primarily centered in the vitreous and/or AC. The cause of the inflammation may be infectious (bacteria or fungi) or noninfectious (e.g., retained lens material or a toxic substance).
- Posterior segment tumor: retinoblastoma or leukemia in children may be associated with AC cell and flare and hypopyon.

- Juvenile xanthogranuloma: children younger than 15 years with raised orange skin lesions. Associated with yellow-gray iris nodules that may spontaneously bleed resulting in hyphema.

■ Diagnostic Evaluation

- Ascertain if there is a history of systemic disease associated with uveitis.
- Complete ophthalmic examination including slit lamp to determine if AC reaction is present and dilated fundus examination to look for signs of vitritis, retinitis, choroiditis, or disc edema. Measure IOP and perform gonioscopy to evaluate the AC angle for peripheral anterior synechia.
- Determine if uveitis is nongranulomatous or granulomatous:
  - Nongranulomatous: fine keratic precipitates on corneal endothelium
  - Granulomatous: large "mutton-fat" keratic precipitates; presence of clusters of cells on the anterior iris surface (Busacca's nodules) or on the pupillary border (Koeppe's nodules). Busacca's nodules are rarely seen in nongranulomatous uveitis.

Note:

- **A patient with a first-time unilateral, nongranulomatous uveitis associated with an unremarkable examination and no significant past medical history is treated for the ocular condition without further systemic workup.**
- **If the uveitis is recurrent, bilateral, or granulomatous (with an unremarkable examination and history), then a nonspecific diagnostic evaluation is pursued.**

Nonspecific Systemic Diagnostic Evaluation

- The following blood tests are performed to determine the cause of the uveitis:
  - Complex blood count (CBC)
  - Erythrocyte sedimentation rate (ESR)
  - Angiotensin-converting enzyme (ACE): elevated in sarcoidosis (but may be low in patient on ACE inhibitors for cardiac conditions)
  - HLA-B27 typing: associated with ankylosing spondylitis, Reiter's syndrome, and HLA-B27-associated uveitis (without systemic disease)
  - FTA-ABS and RPR or VDRL to rule out syphilis
  - Anti-nuclear antibody (ANA) to rule out autoimmune etiology
  - Lyme titer in endemic areas
- Additional tests to consider:
  - PPD and anergy panel
  - Chest x-ray (to rule out TB or sarcoidosis)

- Consider diagnostic vitrectomy with posterior uveitis.
- Consider a CT scan of the brain and a lumbar puncture in human immunodeficiency virus–infected patients because of increased risk of systemic/CNS involvement.

Note: If the history and/or examination suggest a certain cause, then a more specific diagnostic evaluation should be tailored to a more specific diagnosis for the cause of the uveitis.

■ **Treatment**

- Cycloplegic drops (e.g., cyclopentolate 1% to 2%, one drop three times per day) to control pain from iris spasm and to break/prevent posterior synechia.
- Topical steroids (e.g., prednisolone acetate 1%, one drop every 1 to 6 hours) to control inflammation.
- Consider periocular steroid injection (e.g., triamcinolone 20–80 mg) in patients not responding to maximal topical steroids or in posterior uveitis. It is best to wait 4 to 6 weeks on topical steroids before injecting periocular steroid, to determine if the patient is a steroid responder. (See Chapter 8, Steroid Responder Glaucoma.)
- Consider systemic steroids (e.g., prednisone 40–100 mg PO per day) if uveitis is unresponsive to topical or periocular steroid or with posterior uveitis.
- Consider systemic immunosuppressive agents (e.g., cyclosporine or azathioprine) in refractory uveitis.
- Manage elevated IOP created by cellular blockage of the trabecular meshwork, angle closure from peripheral anterior synechia, or steroid responder glaucoma.
  - Use topical beta blocker (e.g., timolol maleate ophthalmic gel forming solution, one drop every day), selective alpha agonists (e.g., brimonidine, one drop twice per day), and topical/systemic carbonic anhydrase inhibitors (e.g., dorzolamide hydrochloride 2%, one drop 2–3 times per day).
  - Do *not* use pilocarpine: may increase inflammation and may result in more elevated IOP because it decreases uveoscleral outflow and the trabecular outflow may already be compromised.
  - Avoid prostaglandin analogs-hypotensive lipids (e.g., latanoprost, bimatoprost, and travoprost) because they may exacerbate inflammation. May use these agents if other glaucoma medications are ineffective and IOP control is urgent and more critical than anti-inflammatory control.
- Medical or rheumatology consult when systemic therapy contemplated.
- Manage systemic cause of uveitis as per internist.

▪ Follow-up

- Patients should be monitored closely for changes in the AC/vitreous reaction.
- Steroid medications should be tapered slowly as AC/vitreous reaction improves.
- IOP measurement to rule out secondary glaucoma.
- Discontinue cycloplegic agent when reaction is resolved.
- Discontinue steroids when no cells visible (may have some flare remaining).
- Discontinue glaucoma medications as IOP improves.
- Monitor for cataract development (especially posterior subcapsular) from chronic steroid use and inflammation.
- Examine patient daily to weekly initially, depending on severity.
- Examine every 1 to 6 months when stable.

10 Retinal and Vitreous Disorders

Angie E. Wen, MD and Thomas E. Bournias, MD

RETINAL ARTERIAL OCCLUSION

Occlusion of the central retinal artery or one of its branches results in ischemia to the retina and subsequent vision loss. The majority of arterial occlusions result from either a thrombotic or an embolic source, and occur mostly in the elderly. In younger patients, retinal artery occlusion is more often associated with migraines, hypercoagulable states, hemoglobinopathies, inflammation, trauma, or congenital disorders of the central retinal artery.

Central Retinal Artery Occlusion (and Branch Retinal Artery Occlusion)

Central retinal artery occlusion (CRAO) occurs at or proximal to the lamina cribrosa. It is more often thrombotic than embolic. A branch retinal artery occlusion (BRAO) may also occur in the superotemporal or inferotemporal arteriole (Plate 15). Two thirds of these cases are secondary to emboli including cholesterol (Hollenhorst plaque), platelet-fibrin, calcific, and septic. Other causes include thrombus, inflammation, hypercoagulable states, and, rarely, giant cell arteritis (GCA).

■ History
- Abrupt, painless, unilateral loss of vision that is often severe (counting fingers to light perception only).
- Amaurosis fugax is a precursor in 10% of CRAOs and 25% of BRAOs.

■ Clinical Manifestations
- Severe loss of vision with a relative afferent pupillary defect (RAPD) in the affected eye.
- Anterior segment examination is usually normal.
- Fundus is initially normal, with ischemic whitening and edema of the retina occurring within hours (Plate 15).

- Cherry-red spot in the center of the macula due to surrounding ischemic whitening.
- Arteriolar narrowing and "boxcar" formation (segmentation of blood column).
- Central vision may be spared if there is a coexistent cilioretinal artery supplying the macula.
- Intact central vision in 50% of BRAOs.
- Emboli (usually Hollenhorst plaque) can be seen in the arterial tree in more than two thirds of cases of BRAO.

■ Etiology

- Thrombosis
- Embolus (usually cardiac or carotid)
- Giant cell arteritis (GCA)
- Collagen vascular disease
  - Systemic lupus erythematosus (SLE)
  - Polyarteritis nodosa
- Hypercoagulable disorders
  - Oral contraceptives
  - Polycythemia
- Trauma
- Migraine

■ Risk Factors

- Hypertension
- Family history
- Atherosclerotic cardiac or carotid disease
- High cholesterol
- Diabetes mellitus
- Smoking
- Oral contraceptives
- Coagulopathies

■ Differential Diagnosis

- Single or multiple branch artery occlusion: retinal changes and loss of vision corresponding to the affected branch artery.
- Ophthalmic artery occlusion: intense whitening of the retina, severe vision loss, and no cherry-red spot.
- Arteritic ischemic optic neuropathy: severe visual loss with an RAPD, optic disc edema, high ESR. Usually older than 50 years.
- Inadvertent intraocular gentamicin injection: retinal ischemia and vision loss; may see diffuse vitreous haze and retinal detachment (RD) (as a result of a toxic amount).
- Cilioretinal artery occlusion: ischemia and whitening in the area of the retina from the disc to the macula. Remaining retina is intact.
- Necrotizing herpetic retinitis: blurry vision, RAPD; painful, cells in vitreous.

- Other causes of a cherry-red spot: often genetic diseases such as Tay-Sachs, bilateral.

■ Diagnostic Evaluation

- Determine the duration of visual loss and if there are coexisting medical conditions.
- Visual acuity and IOP measurement; check pupillary reactions.
- Detailed fundus examination evaluating for retinal ischemia, cherry-red spot.
- Consider fluorescein angiography and/or electroretinography (not helpful in BRAO).
- Check blood pressure.
- Complete blood count, ESR, lipid profile, hypercoagulability panel, serum protein electrophoresis to evaluate for hypercoagulable condition.
- Cardiac echocardiography and color Doppler imaging or carotid ultrasound to look for embolic source.
- Must rule out GCA in all patients older than 50. If ESR is elevated or there is high suspicion, start corticosteroids and perform a temporal artery biopsy.

■ Treatment

- No proven treatments
- Therapies are directed at increasing blood flow, oxygenation, and reversing obstruction (must be performed within 24 hours):
  - Decrease IOP by paracentesis, ocular massage, pharmaceutical agents
  - Anticoagulation
  - Antioxidants
- Corticosteroids (e.g., prednisone 60–100 mg PO daily) in temporal arteritis can help decrease incidence of CRAO in the contralateral eye.
- Panretinal photocoagulation if neovascularization of the retina, disc or iris occurs (occurs in about 20% by one month).
- Anticoagulation in clotting disorders.

■ Follow-up

- Internal medicine consultation for complete workup.
- 1 to 2 weeks initially to monitor for retinal, disc or iris neovascularization.
- If stable after 3 months, follow up every 3–6 months.
- If GCA suspected, perform temporal artery biopsy within 1 to 2 weeks of starting oral steroids.
- Follow up monthly if GCA diagnosed. Taper steroids as symptoms/ESR improve. (ESR is checked monthly.)

Ophthalmic Artery Occlusion

Ophthalmic artery occlusion occurs when there is simultaneous retinal and choroidal circulatory obstruction. This can occur from occlusion at a single site or at multiple sites. Ophthalmic artery occlusion differs from CRAO and BRAO in that there is profound visual acuity loss, usually little to no light perception, and a total afferent pupillary defect (APD). There is also intense whitening of the retina beyond the macula, and little or no cherry-red spot. There is no proven therapy, and significant visual recovery usually does not occur.

RETINAL VEIN OCCLUSION

Central retinal vein occlusion (CRVO) and branch retinal vein occlusion (BRVO) are much more common than retinal artery occlusions. Both occur as a result of impaired venous outflow. CRVO can be ischemic or nonischemic, with a spectrum of clinical presentations. About one third of cases of nonischemic CRVO progress to ischemic within 3 years.

Central Retinal Vein Occlusion (and Branch Retinal Vein Occlusion)

The central retinal artery compresses the central retinal vein in the region of the lamina cribrosa, which results in thrombosis in the vein. This results in a CRVO, causing an increase in the capillary pressure, damage to the endothelium of the vessels, extravasation of blood, and, eventually, hypoxia of the retina. A nonischemic CRVO (75% of cases) occurs when there is leakage from the capillary vessels without nonperfusion. Ischemic CRVO (25% of cases) occurs when there is large area of nonperfusion of the capillaries. A BRVO may occur at an arteriovenous crossing as a result of compression of the vein by a rigid, atherosclerotic artery (Plate 16 and Figure 2-5).

■ **Etiology**

- Atherosclerosis
- Hypertension
- Diabetes mellitus
- Glaucoma (or elevated IOP)
- Optic disc edema or drusen
- Hypercoagulable conditions
  -Polycythemia, multiple myeloma, leukemia

- Vasculitis
  - Systemic lupus erythematosus, sarcoidosis, syphilis
- Abnormal platelet function
- Drugs
  - Birth control pills, diuretics
- Thyroid disease, orbital tumor

■ Epidemiology
- Usually in patients older than 50 years.
- BRVO is three times more common than CRVO.

■ History
- Nonischemic CRVO:
  - Mild to moderate unilateral decrease in visual acuity.
  - Intermittent blurry vision
  - Usually painless
- Ischemic CRVO:
  - Acute, marked unilateral decrease in visual acuity
  - May be painful
- A BRVO may be asymptomatic or result in severe loss of vision.
- A BRVO has a visual field scotoma (blind spot).

■ Clinical Manifestations

Nonischemic CRVO
- Acute or insidious loss of central vision with a slight RAPD
- Dot-and-blot and flame-shaped hemorrhages in all four quadrants of the retina ("blood and thunder")
- Macular edema
- Engorgement and tortuosity of the veins
- Optic nerve swelling with absent venous pulsations (absent in 20% of normals)
- Development of optociliary collateral vessels on the optic nerve over time
- Iris or retinal neovascularization is uncommon

Ischemic CRVO
- Severe visual loss of 20/400 or worse with a prominent RAPD.
- More extensive hemorrhages and engorgement of veins and scattered cotton-wool spots (CWS) (Plate 17).
- Optic disc and macular edema.
- Absent venous pulsations.
- Retinal neovascularization is uncommon.
- Fluorescein angiogram reveals extensive capillary nonperfusion.
- Iris neovascularization in over two thirds of cases.

BRVO (Plate 16 and Figure 2-5)
- Retinal hemorrhages usually do not cross the horizontal raphe (midline).
- Retinal neovascularization in 20%.
- May have associated vitreous hemorrhage.
- Anterior segment neovascularization (i.e., rubeosis iridis) is rare.

■ Risk Factors
- Hypertension
- Diabetes mellitus
- Atherosclerotic cardiovascular disease
- Retinal vasculitis
- Glaucoma or elevated IOP
- Hypercoagulable states
- Trauma

■ Differential Diagnosis
- Ocular ischemic syndrome: dilated veins, retinal hemorrhages primarily in midperiphery and neovascularization of the disc; no optic disc hemorrhages or edema.
- Diabetic retinopathy: microaneurysms and hemorrhages are mostly on the posterior pole. Hard exudates are more common in this condition. Typically bilateral.
- Radiation retinopathy: optic disc edema, CWS, dot-and-blot hemorrhages, and retinal neovascularization primarily in midperiphery; history of radiation therapy.
- Bilateral disc swelling (papilledema) (Plate 7): optic nerve swelling and surrounding flame-shaped hemorrhages do not extend to the peripheral retina. Associated with elevated intracranial pressure.

■ Diagnostic Evaluation
- Determine if there is a history of hypertension, diabetes, or other systemic disease.
- Complete ophthalmologic examination, including dilated retinal examination to rule out macular edema or neovascularization.
- Check blood pressure.
- Fluorescein angiography to rule out macular edema and to assess whether the occlusion is ischemic or nonischemic. There is a greater risk of neovascularization with more capillary nonperfusion.
- Referral to internist for cardiovascular workup (possibly check CBC, fasting glucose level, lipid profile, ESR, hypercoagulability panel).
- An ischemic CRVO tends to be associated with a visual acuity of 20/400 or less, an RAPD, a constricted visual field, and decreased B-wave amplitude on electroretinogram.

■ **Treatment**

- Manage underlying medical conditions.
- Discontinue or change causative medications if possible.
- May try aspirin, anticoagulation, corticosteroids (no proven benefit).
- Reduce IOP if elevated (more than 18 mm Hg) in either eye (see Primary Open Angle Glaucoma in Chapter 8).
- Panretinal photocoagulation if evidence of retinal, optic nerve, or iris neovascularization noted.
- Grid pattern (focal) laser photocoagulation for macular edema.

■ **Follow-up**

- About monthly for first 6 months
- Gonioscopy at each visit to rule out iris neovascularization forming in the anterior chamber angle
- Dilated retinal examination at each visit to watch for macular edema or neovascularization of the retina/disc.

VITREOUS CONDITIONS

Posterior Vitreous Detachment

The vitreous is the transparent gel filling the inner portion of the eyeball between the lens and the retina. Both physiologic changes with advanced age and pathologic processes (e.g., trauma) can disrupt the attachments between the vitreous and retina. Breakdown of the collagen structure causes liquefaction (synersis) of the vitreous and a decrease in gel volume, which predisposes to separation of the vitreous from the retina. A posterior vitreous detachment (PVD) occurs when there is a separation of the vitreous cortex from the retina. A PVD can place traction on the retina, putting a patient at risk for serious complications such as a retinal hole, retinal detachment (RD), and retinal or vitreous hemorrhage.

■ **Epidemiology**

- Present in more than 25% of population by age 40 years
- Present in 60% to 65% of patients by age 80 years

■ **History**

- May be asymptomatic
- Floaters in the form of many shapes (e.g., spiders, cobwebs) that change position with eye movement
- Flashing lights (photopsia) secondary to traction on the retina
- Blurry vision (if floaters present in front of the macula)

■ Clinical Manifestations

- Gray or black opacities from vitreous condensation. These opacities are mobile and change position with eye movement.
- Weiss ring: Previously unseen attachment of the vitreous around the edges of optic nerve that can now be seen suspended and floating in the vicinity of the optic disc (Plate 18).
- Pigmented cells in the anterior vitreous: when associated with an acute PVD, indicates a high possibility of a coexisting retinal tear (Plate 2).
- May see consequences of traction secondary to vitreoretinal adhesions: retinal break or rupture, vitreous or retinal hemorrhage, or RD (Plate 19).

■ Risk Factors

- Advanced age
- Myopia
- Cataract extraction or other eye surgery
- Trauma to the eye

■ Differential Diagnosis

- Migraine: headaches may be accompanied by ocular symptoms including expanding zig-zag lines that may obstruct vision, flashing lights, and dark spots (scintillating scotoma). Ophthalmologic examination is normal.
- Vitritis: inflammatory white cells may be present in the anterior as well as posterior vitreous. Cells are not pigmented. There may be a history of posterior uveitis.
- Retinal break: similar symptoms, pigmented cells may be seen in the vitreous; full-thickness retinal defect may be seen on dilated retinal examination.
- RD: similar symptoms; but elevation of the retina seen on dilated retinal examination.
- Vitreous hemorrhage: may have blurred vision and floaters, visualization of retina may be difficult on dilated retinal examination.

■ Diagnostic Evaluation

- Determine the nature and duration of the flashes/floaters. Distinguish the symptoms of a PVD from the visual changes encountered in a migraine.
- Complete ophthalmologic exam: slit lamp examination to rule out pigmented cells in the anterior vitreous. Dilated retinal examination with scleral depression to look for retinal breaks or an RD.
- B-scan ultrasound to evaluate for an RD or tumor in cases where a vitreous hemorrhage obstructs the view into the back of the eye.

■ Treatment
- No treatment if no sequelae
- Laser photocoagulation or cryotherapy for a new retinal break as soon as possible to prevent RD

■ Follow-up
- Two to four weeks to perform repeat dilated retinal examination. Even after an originally normal retinal examination, a retinal tear or RD can occur several weeks after an acute PVD because the vitreous continues to collapse for a few weeks.
- Sooner if a vitreous or retinal hemorrhage is present.
- Sooner if new or increased flashes/floaters occur.
- Routine follow-up once vitreous has fully detached without evidence of retinal hole or RD.

Vitreous Hemorrhage

Blood in the vitreous usually as a result of bleeding from fragile retinal vessels in proliferative disease (e.g., diabetes), shearing of blood vessels from rapid eye movement or a PVD, or trauma. A vitreous hemorrhage may resolve over several weeks or months, or may require surgical removal with vitrectomy.

■ History
- Painless sudden loss of vision
- Black spots in visual field with possible flashing lights

■ Clinical Manifestations
- Red blood cells in the vitreous
- Obscuring of the retina and retinal vessels by blood
- Mild RAPD
- Loss of "red reflex" in severe vitreous hemorrhage

   Note: If vitreous hemorrhage is present in an infant, consider traumatic child abuse.

■ Etiology
- Diabetic retinopathy
- Retinal detachment/tear
- PVD
- Subarachnoid/subdural hemorrhage (Terson's syndrome)
- Intraocular surgery
- BRVO
- Age-related macular degeneration (AMD)
- Trauma

■ Differential Diagnosis
- Vitritis: onset of symptoms usually less sudden, no hemorrhage is present

- Retinal detahcment (RD): Symptoms are the same as vitreous hemorrhage, but dilated fundus examination reveals an RD with or without an associated vitreous hemorrhage.

■ Diagnostic Evaluation

- Determine if there is a history of trauma or systemic disease.
- Complete ophthalmologic examination including slit lamp to check for neovascularization of the iris (NVI) and retinal examination with scleral depression to rule out a retinal hole or an RD.
- B-scan ultrasound if fundus view is obscured to rule out RD or intraocular tumor.

■ Treatment

- Patients should be closely monitored for signs of RD.
- Aspirin or anticoagulation should be stopped or reversed if not medically necessary.
- Management of predisposing factors (laser or cryotherapy for retinal breaks or retinal vascular diseases; retinopexy or vitrectomy for RDs).
- Pars plana vitrectomy (PPV) if the vitreous hemorrhage is:
  - Associated with an RD or NVI
  - Chronic (more than 6 months duration) or sooner if bilateral
  - Associated with hemolytic or ghost cell glaucoma (but glaucoma procedures may be considered instead)

■ Follow-up

- Every day for 3 days, then every few weeks to months to monitor for reabsorption of the hemorrhage.
- Repeat B-scan ultrasounds may be needed to monitor the hemorrhage and to look for RD if fundus view is impaired.

RETINAL DETACHMENT

An RD occurs when there is a separation of the sensory retina from the retinal pigment epithelium (RPE). Detachments can be rhegmatogenous, exudative, or tractional.

Rhegmatogenous Retinal Detachment

A rhegmatogenous retinal detachment (RRD) occurs in association with a full-thickness defect in the neural retina (retinal break). Liquefied vitreous enters this defect causing a separation of the sensory retina from the RPE (Plate 19). An RRD occurs in 1 in 10,000 individuals.

Exudative Retinal Detachment

An exudative retinal detachment (ERD) is caused by the accumulation of shifting subretinal fluid and subsequent serous elevation of the retina. The processes involved are:

- Increase in flow of vitreous fluid into the subretinal space secondary to damaged RPE
- Impairment of outflow of fluid from the subretinal space
- Impairment of the RPE fluid pump from breakdown of the blood-retina barrier in certain disease states

Tractional Retinal Detachment

Tractional retinal detachment (TRD) results from traction on the retina from rapid eye movements or contraction of fibrous bands that connect the vitreous to the retina.

■ History

- May be asymptomatic
- Central and/or peripheral vision loss
- Flashing lights (photopsias) and/or floaters
- Curtain or shadow in the visual field

■ Clinical Manifestations

RRD

- May have an RAPD or decreased IOP (compared to the contralateral eye)
- Elevation of the retina (with associated retinal break)
- An RRD is often corrugated in appearance with clear subretinal fluid that does not shift with head position (Plate 19).
- Loss of RPE and choroidal detail on retinal examination
- May have pigmented cells in the anterior vitreous (Plate 2)
- May have concurrent PVD or vitreous hemorrhage

ERD

- Smooth elevation of the neural retina above the RPE
- The RD moves with changes in head position
- May find other signs of the causative underlying disease

TRD

- Mild RAPD
- Retina immobile with a smooth, concave elevation

- May find other signs of the causative underlying disease
- May observe vitreous membranes exerting traction on the retina

■ Risk Factors/Causes

RRD
- High myopia
- Previous cataract surgery
- Ocular trauma
- History of PVD
- Cytomegalovirus retinitis
- RD in fellow eye

ERD
- Diabetic retinopathy
- Tumors/neoplasia
- Congenital abnormalities
- Subretinal neovascularization
- Extreme hypertension
- Central serous chorioretinopathy
- Exudative AMD
- Postsurgical complication

TRD
- Proliferative diabetic retinopathy
- Sickle cell hemoglobinopathy
- Retinopathy of prematurity
- Ocular trauma
- Previous RD

■ Differential Diagnosis (any of the above RDs)

- Retinoschisis: splitting of the neural retinal layer. No pigmented cells in the vitreous or retinal hemorrhage. Retina is not mobile with eye movements; often bilateral.
- Choroidal detachment: detachment usually involves the whole periphery of the retina and choroid. It appears more solid with an orange-brown color. No movement with eye motions. The ora serrata may be visible. IOP is often low [less than 6 mm Hg (hypotony)]. Often seen after glaucoma surgery.
- Choroidal tumor: may need to differentiate from retinal/choroidal detachment with ultrasound.
- Vitreous hemorrhage: similar symptoms; preservation of retinal detail seen beyond the hemorrhage.

■ Diagnostic Evaluation

- History and complete ophthalmologic examination with attention to dilated retinal examination with scleral depression; look for retinal break to rule out RRD
- B-scan ultrasound, if view is obscured with vitreous hemorrhage or to look for subretinal fluid shifts with head position
- With ERD: CT or MRI to rule out tumors/masses

■ **Treatment**
- Goal is to reestablish contact between the RPE and the sensory retina.
- RRD/TRD: laser photocoagulation, pneumatic retinopexy, cryopexy, PPV, scleral buckle.
- ERD: treatment is directed at the underlying cause. Laser photocoagulation, cryotherapy, or diathermy for peripheral vascular lesions. Radiation therapy for ocular tumors.

■ **Follow-up**
- For RRD/TRD, immediate repair if fovea is involved; otherwise as soon as possible.
- For ERD, depends on the primary disease process. There is often recovery of vision with resolution of excess subretinal fluid.

AGE-RELATED MACULAR DEGENERATION

Age-related macular degeneration (AMD) is a degenerative disease in which there is gradual loss of central vision as a result of nutrient and oxygen deprivation of the retinal tissue. There are two main forms: nonexudative (or dry) (Plate 20) and exudative (or wet) (Plate 21). Although visual loss is more severe in wet AMD, there are proven treatments for some types of wet AMD whereas no definitive therapy exists for dry AMD.

■ **Pathogenesis**
- Exact cause is poorly understood.
- Visual loss is secondary to RPE/retinal atrophy, RPE detachment, and choroidal neovascularization.

■ **Epidemiology**
- Most common cause of severe central vision loss in people older than 50 years in developed countries
- Incidence increases with age
- Much more common in lighter pigmental individuals (i.e., whites, blue-eyed individuals)

■ **History**
- Progressive, painless loss of central vision
- Distortion of images (metamorphopsia)
- May be asymptomatic

■ Clinical Manifestations

Nonexudative AMD

- Geographic chorioretinal atrophy: atrophy of the RPE that often coalesces into a ring or petalloid pattern around the fovea
- Hyper- or hypopigmentation in the RPE
- Drusen: focal whitish yellow excrescences under the retina [at the level of the RPE and Bruch's membrane (Plate 20)]
- RPE detachment

Exudative AMD

In addition to the above signs, may also see:

- Choroidal neovascularization (CNV): growth of blood vessels from the choriocapillaris that break through Bruch's membrane and gain entry into the subretinal space [usually the macular area (Plate 21)]
- Subretinal fluid, hemorrhage, and exudates
- Macular edema
- Disciform scarring (subretinal fibrosis)
- Vitreous/retinal hemorrhage

■ Possible Risk Factors

- Advanced age
- Atherosclerosis
- Light/solar damage
- Vitamin and essential element deficiencies
- High risk for subsequent CNV:
  - Multiple large (more than 64 μm) drusen
  - Focal RPE hyperpigmentation
- Risk of CNV is 10% to 12% per year if contralateral eye involved
- Genetics (family and personal history)
- Hypertension
- Smoking
- Hyperopia

■ Differential Diagnosis

- Hereditary diseases (pattern dystrophy, Best's disease, Stargardt's disease, angioid streaks)
- Degenerative myopia: macular and optic disc changes without drusen
- Central serous chorioretinopathy: retinal elevation, atrophy and detachment of the RPE; no drusen or subretinal blood, usually seen in younger patients
- Multifocal choroiditis: chorioretinal atrophy without drusen
- Toxic lesions secondary to drug exposure: variable hyper- and hypopigmentation; no drusen (e.g., chloroquine toxicity with its characteristic "bull's eye" maculopathy)

- Ocular histoplasmosis: whitish yellow chorioretinal lesions with distorted vision; younger patients; no drusen; and atrophy near the optic disc is usually present
- Choroidal osteoma: yellowish orange geographic lesions with retinal degeneration; a benign tumor of dense bone detectable on B-scan ultrasonography
- Angioid streaks: lesions are gray or reddish brown and are arranged around the optic disc
- Sarcoidosis: precipitates are present on the cornea; iritis and vitritis often seen
- Choroidal rupture: yellow-white subretinal streaks; usually are located near the disc and associated with trauma
- Other causes of subretinal hemorrhage or fluid

■ Diagnostic Evaluation

- History and complete ophthalmologic examination: key features are geographic chorioretinal atrophy, RPE detachment, CNV
- Amsler grid testing to look for metamorphopsia and to detect loss of vision in central 20 degrees of field (paracentral scotoma)
- Fluorescein angiography to determine location of possible CNV lesion, especially when visual acuity has declined or an RPE detachment has occurred.
- Indocyanine green angiographic examination for occult CNV

■ Treatment

- Nonexudative AMD:
  - No proven treatment for visual loss.
  - Antioxidants and zinc (e.g., Ocuvite and I-Caps) have been shown to slow progression.
- Exudative AMD:
  - Laser photocoagulation for well-defined CNV only (15% to 20% of cases).
  - Photodynamic therapy (PDT): better outcomes early in the disease where lesions are small. This procedure has slowed the loss of vision in some, and only rarely improves visual activity.
  - Surgery to remove subretinal CNV has had limited success because of loss of RPE associated with extraction of the neovascular membrane. Surgery involving plication of the outer sclera and retinal rotation has also demonstrated limited success. Patients often need subsequent strabismus surgery because of rotational effects generated by altering the location of the macula in these procedures.

-The utilization of surgical procedures has been drastically reduced since PDT was introduced.

-Recent clinical trials have demonstrated less severe loss of vision with intravitreal injections of inhibitors of vascular endothelial growth factor (anti-VEGF).

■ Follow-up

- Nonexudative AMD and poorly defined exudative AMD: 3 to 6 months (looking for signs of a CNV).
- Post-laser treatment for well-defined AMD: 1 month, 3 months, then every 3 to 6 months.
- Patients should use an Amsler grid daily.
- Low vision therapy/consult in patients with bilateral poor vision.

11

Systemic Disorders with Ocular Manifestations

Anthony Cirino, MD and Thomas E. Bournias, MD

Hypertension

Hypertension is a risk factor for heart disease, renal insufficiency, stroke, and vision loss. Uncontrolled hypertension results in a higher risk of retinal vascular changes. The exact pathophysiologic process of hypertensive damage to the retina (hypertensive retinopathy) is not known, but it results in closure of the retinal microvasculature. This retinopathy can resemble other vascular diseases such as diabetes. The incidence of hypertensive retinopathy in hypertensive patients without coexisting vascular diseases is 15%.

■ History

- Relatively asymptomatic disease that rarely produces visual symptoms
- Scotomas: can occasionally result from more advanced disease such as large retinal hemorrhages, cotton-wool spots, or retinal vascular occlusive diseases such as retinal vein occlusion or ischemic optic neuropathy
- Diplopia: ischemia to nerves that control the extraocular muscles (EOMs) resulting in symptoms
  - Motility function usually returns to normal in weeks to months.
  - Most commonly CN VI and IV, and occasionally III.

■ Clinical Manifestation

- Most common findings are focal constriction and dilation of retinal arterioles.
- Increased tortuosity of retinal vessels.
- Hallmark is arteriovenous nicking (AVN).
- Copper wiring: narrowed vessels.
- Silver wiring: occluded vessels.
- Cotton-wool spots: infarcts of ganglion cell axons (Plate 17).
- Retinal hemorrhages including microaneurysms, dot-and-blot hemorrhages, and flame-shaped hemorrhages. Blood or exudate forms round blots in the middle and outer layers of the

retina where small capillaries are found and the overall direction of the cells is perpendicular to the plane of the retinal pigment epithelium. Flame-shaped hemorrhages occur in the inner retina where the nerve fiber layer is parallel to the retinal surface (see Figure 1-7).

- Hard exudates: exudation of lipoproteins. Hard exudates may coalesce in the macula resulting in a macular star (Plate 8). This occurs because at the fovea the outer layers of the retina tend to be parallel to the surface (Henle's layer) and any material (including hard exudates) in these extracellular spaces results in radial or star-shaped patterns.
- Ocular complications include retinal vascular occlusive disease, macroaneurysms, and nonarteritic ischemic optic neuropathies.
- Macular edema in advanced cases (Plate 8).
- If malignant hypertension (250 mm Hg systolic and 150 mm Hg diastolic):
  - Papilledema, superficial retinal hemorrhages (Plate 8).
  - Medical emergency: prompt medical attention to prevent serious complications including myocardial infarction, stroke, kidney failure, and encephalopathy.
  - Untreated mortality rate is 50% at 2 months and 90% at 1 year.

■ **Differential Diagnosis (of hypertensive retinopathy)**

- Age-related atherosclerotic changes: no associated systemic hypertension.
- Diabetic retinopathy (DR): develops neovascularization, microaneurysms, and dot-and-blot hemorrhages without significant retinal vessel narrowing.
- Anemia: no associated hypertension; hemorrhages may occur, but usually no significant arterial changes.
- Venous occlusions, such as central retinal vein occlusion (CRVO) or branch retinal vein occlusion (BRVO): dilated, tortuous veins with adjacent retinal hemorrhages; usually unilateral.
- Collagen vascular diseases: retinal findings are usually primarily cotton-wool spots only.
- Human immunodeficiency virus (HIV) retinopathy: history of HIV infection.
- Ocular ischemic syndrome: usually demonstrates dot-and-blot hemorrhages in the midperipheral retina in all four quadrants. May have amaurosis fugax or ocular pain.
- Radiation retinopathy: usually associated with a history of irradiation to the head area. Retinal changes are similar to hypertensive retinopathy but usually develop after one year or more of irradiation.

■ Risk Factors

- Diabetes mellitus
- Smoking
- Sedentary life style, obesity
- Hereditary factors
- Preeclampsia in previous pregnancies

■ Diagnostic Evaluation

- Ascertain if there is a history of hypertension/diabetes or radiation therapy.
- Check blood pressure.
- Dilated fundus examination to inspect the retina for vascular changes or hemorrhage

■ Treatment

- Blood pressure control.
- Referral to a primary care physician. However, immediate referral to the emergency room is recommended if the diastolic blood pressure is greater than 110 mm Hg, there is chest pain or difficulty breathing, there are mental status changes or headache, or there is decreased vision with disc edema.
- Chronic changes produced by hypertension will not resolve.

■ Follow-up

- Minimal hypertensive retinopathy and controlled blood pressure requires only annual examination
- More severe hypertensive retinopathy requires more frequent examinations

Diabetes Mellitus

The exact mechanism by which diabetes causes retinopathy remains unclear. It results in microaneurysms, which leak plasma components into the retina causing edema and hard exudates. In addition, microvascular occlusion, capillary dropout and neovascularization (growth of abnormal vessels in a hypoxic retina) may occur. Clinically, there are two main types of diabetic retinopathy (DR): nonproliferative (NPDR or background) and proliferative (PDR).

■ Epidemiology

- Prevalence of diabetic retinopathy in insulin-dependent diabetes mellitus is 40% compared to 20% in non–insulin-dependent diabetes mellitus.
- Some form of DR is present in 90% of patients who have had diabetes for 17–25 years.
- DR is the most common cause of legal blindness in individuals aged 20 to 65.

■ **History**
- Early changes in NPDR are most often asymptomatic.
- Decreased vision due to any of the following:
  - Clinically significant macular edema (CSME)
  - Vitreous hemorrhage
  - Ischemia to the macula

■ **Clinical Manifestation**
- Ophthalmic complications include DR (NPDR and PDR), corneal abnormalities, glaucoma (POAG or neovascular), iris neovascularization, cataracts, and cranial nerve palsies (usually III, IV or VI).

Nonproliferative Diabetic Retinopathy (Plate 22)
- Usually bilateral and more prominent on the posterior pole
- Microaneurysms (dot): first detected clinically
- Intraretinal hemorrhages (blot)
- Hard exudates: waxy yellow deposits often associated with edema
- Retinal edema
- Cotton-wool spots (Plate 17)
- Intraretinal microvascular abnormalities: preproliferative

Proliferative Diabetic Retinopathy
- Neovascularization is the hallmark of PDR (Plate 23).
- Neovascularization can occur in the retina, optic nerve, iris, or anterior chamber angle.
- Can result in fibrovascular proliferation leading to traction retinal detachment (TRD).
- Vitreous hemorrhage can occur causing acute vision loss.

Diabetic Maculopathy (clinically significant macular edema)
- Most common cause of visual impairment
- Macular thickening due to leaking vessels: diffuse or focal
- Hard exudates
- Ischemia resulting in poor vision

■ **Risk Factors**
- Duration of diabetes: most important factor.
  - DM type I: DR rare after 5 years, but 90% have DR after 30 years.
  - DM type II: 5% have DR at presentation.
- Poor blood sugar control results in worse DR.
- Pregnancy.
- Hypertension.
- Renal disease.
- Corticosteroid use.
- Others: obesity, hypercholesterolemia, smoking, anemia.

■ Differential Diagnosis

Nonproliferative Diabetic Retinopathy
- HIV retinopathy: glucose normal, more cotton-wool spots
- Ocular ischemic syndrome: glucose normal, narrowed vessels, hemorrhages diffuse throughout retina
- Hypertensive retinopathy: high blood pressure, narrowed retinal vessels
- Emboli from intravenous drug abuse

Proliferative Diabetic Retinopathy (PDR)
- Retinal venous occlusion (e.g., CRVO or BRVO): dilated, tortuous vessels
- Sickle cell retinopathy: usually in retinal periphery, history of sickle cell disease or trait
- Ocular ischemic syndrome
- Emboli from intravenous drug abuse: may result in peripheral retinal neovascularization

■ Diagnostic Evaluation
- Random glucose level and hemoglobin A_{1c}.
- Ophthalmic examination: slit lamp examination to detect neovascularization of the iris. Gonioscopy to detect neovascularization in the anterior chamber angle. Dilated fundus examination to detect CSME, disc neovascularization, or retinal neovascularization.
- Fluorescein angiography may be helpful.

■ Treatment

Nonproliferative Diabetic Retinopathy
- Observation
- Better control of blood glucose, blood pressure, anemia, and renal failure

Proliferative Diabetic Retinopathy
- Panretinal photocoagulation, especially if neovascularization of the iris is present.
- Consider peripheral retinal cryotherapy if there is not an adequate view of the fundus and traction on the retina is not present.
- Pars plana vitrectomy for chronic vitreous hemorrhage.
- Retinal detachment repair if present.

Clinically Significant Macular Edema (CSME)
- Focal laser photocoagulation to microaneurysms.
- Corticosteroid injection (intravitreal) may be considered.

Glaucoma
- POAG: Treat IOP as per Chapter 8
- Neovascular glaucoma (NVG)
  -PRP as soon as possible.
  -IOP is difficult to control and often requires interventional therapy with TSCP (diode) or aqueous shunt.

Carnial Nerve Palsy
- No treatment, usually resolves within 3 months
- Often associated with pain
- CN III palsy spares the pupil (i.e., no dilation)

■ Follow-up
- No DR: annual examination
- Mild-moderate NPDR: every 6 months
- Severe NPDR: every 2 to 6 months
- PDR: dilated fundus examination every 2 to 4 months or more frequent depending on severity

Multiple Sclerosis

Multiple sclerosis (MS) is an inflammatory demyelinating condition of the central nervous system (CNS) affecting the white matter of the brain, the spinal cord, and the optic nerves. Affected tissues demonstrate infiltration by lymphocytes and monocytes. The pathophysiologic process is not completely known, but it has been suggested that the immune system is triggered to attack the host. This trigger is not known, but a viral cause has been suggested.

■ Epidemiology
- Most prevalent in whites of northern European descent and in persons living in temperate climates.
- Both genetic and environmental factors influence the frequency.
- Prevalence in the United States is approximately 1 in 1000.
- Affects women more than men (about 2:1 in many series).

■ History
- Variable degrees of fatigue and exhaustion
- Fatigue after taking a hot shower or after intense exercise
- Heat-induced episodes of optic nerve dysfunction termed Uhthoff's phenomenon
- Sudden and gradual visual loss described as patchy or dark areas in their vision, color or brightness reduction, photopsias, or mild blurred vision
- Double vision, pain with eye movement

■ Clinical Manifestation

- Varied clinical course with distinct classifications
- Cognitive changes, hemiparesis, ataxia, depression, or visual symptoms
- Diplopia (double vision) in 10%
- Nystagmus in 35%
- Internuclear ophthalmoplegia (INO) (11%)
  - Lesion of the medial longitudinal fasciculus
  - Impaired adduction of the ipsilateral eye with lateral gaze nystagmus of the contralateral eye
  - Bilateral INO considered pathognomonic of MS
- Optic neuritis: clinical triad of loss of vision, eye pain, and dyschromatopsia (impairment of color vision)
  - 20% of all patients with definite MS initially present with optic neuritis.
  - Unilateral in 70% of cases.
  - Pain behind eye worse with eye movement.
  - Majority of optic neuritis is retrobulbar (behind the globe) with the optic disc appearing normal clinically.

■ Risk Factors

- Female
- Age 20 to 40 (mean age of onset 30 years)
- Family history of MS
- HLA-DR2 haplotype
- Whites of Scandinavian or North Sea ancestry
- Environmental influences
- Living further from the equator

■ Differential Diagnosis

- Ischemic optic neuropathy: altitudinal defects more common, hemorrhages more common
- Infiltrative nerve process: more gradual onset of symptoms
- Graves' disease: associated proptosis, lid retraction is usually present
- Intraorbital/intracranial compressive lesions: more gradual onset of symptoms
- Miscellaneous inflammatory/infectious and toxic optic neuropathies: rarely pain on eye movement
- Retinal pathology: differentiated by dilated fundus exam

■ Diagnostic Evaluation

- Check vision and the presence of a relative afferent pupillary defect (RAPD).
- Dilated fundus examination to rule out vitritis and to evaluate the optic nerve for hyperemia and blurred disc margins with hemorrhages.

- Test ocular motility, color vision, and confrontational visual fields.
- Visual field testing: Goldmann or Humphry.
- MRI to evaluate the brain and optic nerve:
  - MRI with lesions of high T2 signal intensity of variable location in the white matter of the brain, brain stem, optic nerves, or spinal cord are seen in MS.
  - MRI lesions do not always correlate with clinical symptoms.
  - Patients with optic neuritis and normal brain MRI: studies suggest that 0% to 5% develop clinically definite MS compared to 30% to 50% of patients with three or more periventricular or ovoid white matter lesions.
- Lumbar puncture: 85% of patients have oligoclonal bands in the cerebrospinal fluid.
- Miscellaneous laboratory tests include CBC, PPD antigen, Lyme titers, ESR, ANA, and FTA-ABS/VDRL.

■ Treatment

- Optic neuritis: Intravenous corticosteroid therapy can accelerate short-term vision recovery but does not alter final visual outcome.
- Steroids do not prevent MS.
- Recently, intramuscular interferon β_{1a} therapy initiated during a first demyelinating event (including optic neuritis) has been shown to decrease the likelihood of progression to clinically definite MS.
- Visual outcome is good for most patients.
- Early treatment is essential.

■ Follow-up

- Followed by neurologist and ophthalmologist.
- Patients with MS commonly have acute exacerbations, including optic neuritis.
- Ophthalmologic follow-up includes monitoring of visual acuity, color vision, and visual field.

Thyroid Eye Disease

Thyroid eye disease encompasses a clinical spectrum called thyroid-associated ophthalmopathy (TAO) or Graves' disease. There is an autoimmune-mediated inflammation of the EOMs and orbital and periorbital tissues with resultant infiltration of lymphocytes and glycosaminoglycans. This results in osmotic damage leading to proptosis, fibrosis, and eventually tissue atrophy.

■ Epidemiology

- TAO in the United States has been estimated to have an incidence rate of 16 cases per 100,000 women and 2.9 cases per 100,000 men.

- It affects women 2.5 to 6 times more frequently than men.
- TAO mostly affects patients between the ages of 30 to 50 years.

■ History

- Patients can have dry eyes, foreign body sensation and chemosis, puffy eyelids, "angry-looking eyes," bulging eyes, diplopia, visual loss, visual field loss, ocular pressure or pain, and dyschromatopsia.
- May develop tremor, weight loss, hair loss, goiter, and irritability.
- TAO is the most common cause of unilateral *and* bilateral proptosis in adults.
- Proptosis occurs when the orbital contents expand beyond their normal volume. Since the orbit is made of bone, the only direction in which the globe can decompress is anteriorly.
- Symptoms of an associated hyperthyroidism include tachycardia, nervousness, and diaphoresis.
- Symptoms of hypothyroidism include bradycardia, drowsiness, poor mentation, weight gain, dry skin, depression, cold intolerance, and husky voice.
- TAO may occur in hyperthyroid, hypothyroid, or euthyroid states.

■ Clinical Manifestation

- Dry eyes: redness on conjunctiva and over muscle insertions, chemosis (conjunctival swelling), punctate corneal staining with fluorescein.
- Upper lid retraction due to proptosis, sympathetic drive of Müller's muscle, upgaze restriction, and fibrosis of the levator muscle.
- Lid lag: when patient looks slowly from upgaze to downgaze, eyelids lag behind the globe.
- Diplopia: restrictive myopathy of EOMs resulting in strabismus.
- Visual loss, dyschromatopsia, or visual field loss may indicate compressive optic neuropathy.

■ Risk Factors

- Smoking
- Other autoimmune diseases, such as myasthenia gravis.
- Addison's disease, vitiligo, and pernicious anemia have been associated with TAO.

■ Differential Diagnosis

Conditions that cause proptosis are as follows:

- Cellulitis (orbital and preseptal): acute onset, tenderness, erythema to eyelids; may have associated sinus infection or lid abrasion.

- Orbital masses: proptosis is more gradual. May detect mass with imaging.
- Orbital inflammatory disease (orbital pseudotumor): acute onset of symptoms; often associated with pain.
- Cavernous sinus thrombosis: presents with signs similar to orbital cellulitis with multiple cranial nerve paresis. Usually bilateral with rapid progression. May be associated with nausea and vomiting.
- Carotid cavernous fistula: often with elevated intraocular pressure; history of trauma or surgery but may occur spontaneously. The patient may notice a bruit.
- Pseudoproptosis: enophthalmos of the contralateral eye (e.g., orbital floor fracture). Myopic eyes may be large and associated with tilted discs and peripapillary crescents.

■ Diagnostic Evaluation

- Determine the rapidity of onset of symptoms and if associated with pain. Ascertain if there is a history of systemic disease that can be associated with proptosis or EOM restriction such as diabetes, cancer, or lung disease. Determine if there is a history of trauma.
- Consider TAO in patients with dry eyes, diplopia, or proptosis.
- Check visual acuity, color vision, and the presence or absence of a relative afferent pupillary defect (RAPD) to verify that there is no retrobulbar compression of the optic nerve.
- Measure eyelid position. Determine the degree of proptosis using an exophthalmometer.
- Check extraocular muscle motility for any misalignment. If an abnormality is discovered with an EOM, perform forced duction testing to determine if there is a restriction.
- Measure any ocular misalignment with prisms.
- Digital palpation of the globes is a useful test that can reveal decreased orbital retropulsion.
- Check IOP and visual field.
- Dilated examination to check the optic nerve for signs of swelling.
- Thyroid function tests [thyroid-stimulating hormone (TSH) and free thyroxine (T_4)].
- Neuroimaging usually reveals thickened muscle bodies with tendon sparing. A dilated superior ophthalmic vein may also be present.
- MRI is more sensitive for showing optic nerve compression, whereas CT scanning is performed prior to orbital decompression surgery.

■ Treatment

- Internist or endocrinologist to manage systemic disease.
- There is no immediate cure. Most patients can be observed with management of symptoms only.
- Regulation of thyroid function does not stop or decrease orbital involvement. However, restoration of the euthyroid state (with antithyroid drugs and thyroxine) may improve the eye status to some extent.
- If a patient has dry-eye symptoms, consider using artificial tears during the day, lubricating ointment at night, and punctal plugs. May also tape eyelids closed at night to manage exposure keratopathy.
- Encourage patients to stop smoking to decrease the risk of congestive orbitopathy.
- Symptoms of stable diplopia can be managed with prisms in the spectacle lenses; occasionally muscle surgery may be necessary.
- If compressive optic neuropathy is present, treatment includes immediate administration of oral steroids (e.g., prednisone 100 mg PO every day) or orbital irradiation (to avoid steroids).
- If no visual improvement with steroids or radiation is noted within 2 to 7 days, orbital decompression surgery should be performed.
- If necessary, orbital decompression surgery may be followed by strabismus surgery, then eyelid surgery.

■ Follow-up

- Monitor for vision loss from corneal exposure and optic neuropathy and for strabismus development.
- Visual field and color vision testing may help in early detection of visual loss.
- Frequency depends on severity of symptoms.
- If fluctuating diplopia and/or ptosis, consider myasthenia gravis workup (e.g., Tensilon Test).

Pregnancy

Many physiologic changes affect the body during pregnancy, including the eyes. Both normal and pathologic ocular conditions occur.

■ History

- One of the most common visual symptoms during pregnancy is blurry vision. However, the symptoms can vary in relation to the pathologic process.
- Other symptoms include photopsias, scotomas, diplopia, and headache.

■ Clinical Manifestation

- Physiologic changes: increased pigmentation around the eyes and cheeks (chloasma), decreased corneal sensitivity (possibly necessitating the temporary discontinuation of contact lens use because of an increased risk of infection), and changes in corneal curvature or accomodation resulting in blurry vision. These changes generally resolve after pregnancy.
- Pregnancy-induced hypertensive retinopathy (preeclampsia)
  - Ocular sequelae in up to one third of cases.
  - Patients may develop retinopathy (manifestation similar to hypertensive retinopathy, see hypertension above), optic neuropathy, serous retinal detachments, and occipital cortical changes.
- Toxemia of pregnancy and/or disseminated intravascular coagulation can occur resulting in vascular infarction presenting as a serous retinal detachment.
- Occlusive vascular disorders due to a hypercoagulable state, such as the development of retinal artery and vein occlusion, amniotic fluid embolism, and cerebral venous thrombosis.
- Progression of diabetic retinopathy (DR):
  - Approximately 10% of pregnant diabetic women with no non-proliferative retinopathy or mild nonproliferative retinopathy at the onset of pregnancy will progress.
  - Up to 50% of patients who had moderate or high risk (cotton-wool spots, venous beading, intraretinal microvascular abnormalities) nonproliferative DR show an increase in their retinopathy. This often improves after delivery.
  - Up to 25% of pregnant diabetic women with proliferative retinopathy (PDR) at the onset of pregnancy will progress.
- Other retinal pathology includes: central serous chorioretinopathy and Purtcher's retinopathy.
- Intracerebral and other tumors:
  - Previously asymptomatic pituitary adenomas or microadenomas may enlarge and result in various ophthalmic symptoms, such as headache, visual field change (classically a bitemporal hemianopia), and/or visual acuity loss. Pituitary apoplexy (a potentially life-threatening event) must be ruled out in any pregnant woman with a pituitary adenoma who complains of headache or a new visual field defect. A brain MRI with or without lumbar puncture should be performed to rule out subarachnoid hemorrhage.
  - Meningiomas are benign, slow-growing tumors that may develop very aggressive growth patterns. These are difficult to treat in pregnancy.

- Other causes of headache include: migraine (worse during and immediately postpartum) and pseudotumor cerebri.

■ Risk Factors
- Previous ocular disease or previous ocular pathologic process during a pregnancy
- Systemic diseases (e.g., diabetes mellitus, hypertension)

■ Diagnostic Evaluation
- Ophthalmic examination, including dilated fundus exam, for patients with known diabetes
- Visual field testing in selected patients
- Neuroimaging in patients with visual field defects or scotomas

■ Treatment
- Based on clinical findings and individual diseases.
- Delivery can often limit or resolve ophthalmic manifestations.
- Observation is often the best course.
- PDR requires laser photocoagulation therapy.

■ Follow-up
- Determined by severity of ocular disease.
  - Gestational diabetes only: no follow-up
  - Mild nonproliferative retinopathy: examine in first and third trimester
  - Moderate nonproliferative diabetic retinopathy: examine every trimester
  - High risk nonproliferative retinopathy: examine every month
  - Proliferative retinopathy: examine monthly and treat with laser panretinal photocoagulation
- It is recommended that pregnant patients with pituitary adenomas and microadenomas have monthly ophthalmic follow-up care with visual field assessment to rule out enlargement.

Syphilis

Exposure to the exclusively human pathogen *Treponema pallidum* results in syphilis. It may be congenital (transplacental transmission) or acquired (sexual transmission).

■ Epidemiology
- Occurrence higher in urban populations
- Increased incidence in AIDS patients
- Higher incidence in males than in females

■ **History**
- Blurry vision, photophobia, eye redness
- Diplopia
- Visual field changes caused by gummatous involvement of the brain

■ **Clinical Manifestation**

Congenital Syphilis
Manifestations of the disease affect approximately 70% of infected newborn infants, including:

- Acute and chronic iritis: AC cell and flare.
- Interstitial keratitis: cellular infiltration with superficial and deep vascularization of the cornea. Usually occurs acutely by age 20 years with both eyes becoming involved. Ghost vessels (blood vessels without blood) may develop in the cornea as the inflammation resolves.
- Scleritis, secondary cataract.
- Chorioretinitis ("salt and pepper" fundus): retina contains pigmented areas interspersed with atrophic white areas.
- Optic neuritis or optic nerve pallor (atrophy).

Acquired Syphilis
Three stages: primary, secondary, and tertiary

1. Primary syphilis
   -Painless ulcer on the conjunctiva (chancre), eyelid, or skin 9 to 90 days after exposure; regional lymphadenopathy
2. Secondary syphilis
   -Mucocutaneous involvement: rash on trunk, palms, soles after 8 weeks or more. May have general lymphadenopathy and constitutional symptoms.
   -10% with ocular involvement including: conjunctivitis, episcleritis/scleritis, interstitial keratitis, uveitis, retinitis, choroiditis, retinal vasculitis, optic neuritis, and dacroadenitis.
3. Tertiary syphilis
   -30% of untreated patients. Develops 5 to 30 years from time of infection.
   -Argyll Robertson pupil (see Chapter 6, p. 66), interstitial keratitis, chronic iritis, old chorioretinitis, and optic atrophy.
   -Aortitis, neurosyphilis, others.

- Can mimic many other ocular disorders—the "great imitator"
- Latent stage is usually without clinical manifestations.

■ **Risk Factors**
- Unprotected sexual activity
- Intravenous drug abuse
- Immunocompromised (e.g., AIDS)

■ Differential Diagnosis

Conditions often associated with uveitis:

• Congenital infections, such as toxoplasmosis, herpes simplex or zoster virus, rubella, cytomegalovirus, rubeola (measles)
• Uveitis: idiopathic, sarcoidosis
• HIV: uveitis not typical, HIV testing often necessary
• Tuberculosis: can look similar, but FTA-ABS is negative
• Many others depending on presentation including: Lyme disease, Behçet's disease, HLA-B27 associated conditions, Reiter's syndrome, juvenile rheumatoid arthritis

■ Diagnostic Evaluation

• Obtain detailed sexual history and evidence of previous treatment for syphilis.
• Complete ophthalmic exam including pupils, slit lamp, and dilated fundus exam.
• FTA-ABS test specific to detect antitreponemal antibodies.
• VDRL/RPR: nonspecific tests for screening.
  -False positives in infectious mononucleosis, mycoplasma, malaria, systemic lupus erythematosus (SLE)
• MHA-TP and TPHA (hemagglutination tests for *Treponema pallidum*): specific, but may be negative in early syphilis.
• Uveitis workup includes both FTA-ABS and VDRL.
• HIV testing due to comorbidity of diseases.
• Lumbar puncture (especially if chorioretinitis or papillitis is present) to evaluate for neurosyphilis.
• Neuroretinitis is diagnostic for neurosyphilis.

Note: Patients with concurrent HIV and active syphilis may have negative serologies (RPR, FTA-ABS) because of their immunocompromised state.

■ Treatment

• Patients with ocular syphilis are treated the same as those with neurosyphilis.
• Treatment indications:
  -No treatment if FTA-ABS is negative.
  -Treat if FTA-ABS positive and VDRL negative and appropriate previous treatment cannot be documented.
  -Treat if FTA-ABS positive and VDRL positive and appropriate previous treatment cannot be documented or previous treatment did not result in a fourfold decrease in VDRL titer.
  -May need to treat despite past treatment or VDRL if there are signs of active syphilis (e.g., papillitis, chorioretinitis).
• Treat with penicillin G (e.g., 50,000 u/kg/day, IM or IV in two divided doses) for 10 to 14 days.

- Alternatives (for penicillin-allergic patients) include oral tetracycline (e.g., 500 mg PO four times per day for 30 days) or erythromycin (e.g., 50 mg/kg/day PO in four divided doses) for 2 weeks.
- Treat sexual partners.
- Treat for possible *Chlamydia* infection (e.g., tetracycline, doxycycline, erythromycin) for 3 to 6 weeks.
- Manage uveitis or interstitial keratitis with topical cycloplegics and steroids (e.g., prednisolone acetate, one drop 4 to 8 times per day).
- Manage elevated IOP/glaucoma preferably with topical beta blockers, alpha adrenergics, and topical/oral carbonic anhydrase inhibitors.
- Penetrating keratoplasty (corneal transplant) for corneal scarring from keratitis.

■ Follow-up
- Monitor titers for evidence of response or treatment failures.
- Frequent ocular examinations to monitor resolution of inflammation and control of IOP.
- Often full visual recovery if treated early.
- If patient is untreated, secondary glaucoma, chronic vitritis, retinal necrosis, and optic atrophy may develop.
- If neurosyphilis, every 6 months with lumbar puncture for 2 years.

Stevens-Johnson Syndrome (Erythema Multiforme Major)

An immune complex–mediated hypersensitivity disorder (type III). There are four etiologic categories of Stevens-Johnson syndrome: (1) infectious, (2) drug induced, (3) malignancy related, and (4) idiopathic.

Fifty percent of cases are idiopathic. Common precipitating drugs include penicillins, sulfas, phenytoin (and related anticonvulsants), carbamazepine, and barbiturates. Common infectious agents include various bacteria (especially *Mycoplasma*) and viruses (especially herpes) and fungi.

■ Epidemiology
- Predominantly in whites
- Most common in second to fourth decade
- Blindness secondary to severe keratitis or panophthalmitis in 3% to 10% of patients

■ History
- Following exposure to medications
- Acute onset of fever, skin rash, ocular redness, discharge, foreign body sensation, decreased vision
- Often accompanied by arthralgia and malaise

■ Clinical Manifestation
- Skin may contain "target lesions" and vesicles, bullae, and maculopapular lesions primarily on the hands and feet.
- Mucosal pseudomembrane formation may lead to mucosal scarring, especially of the mouth, lips, and conjunctiva.
- May develop dry eye and symblepharon (conjunctival scarring).
- Cornea may develop neovascularization, scarring, ulcers, and perforation.
- May develop eyelid deformities including trichiasis.

■ Risk Factors
- Drugs and malignancies most often are implicated.
- Pediatric cases are related more often to infections.
- Exposure to inciting agents above.

■ Differential Diagnosis
Conditions resulting in bilateral slow, progressive conjunctival scarring with symblepharon, shortening of the fornices, and dry eye include:
- Ocular cicatricial pemphigoid
- Others including: topical medications, burns (thermal or chemical), recent surgery

■ Diagnostic Evaluation
- Based on history and clinical presentation to determine the precipitating factor
- Ocular examination to evaluate for conjunctival scarring (evert the eyelids)
- Conjunctival and corneal scrapings for stains/cultures (to determine infectious cause if suspected)
- Blood work including CBC, electrolytes

■ Treatment
- Hospitalization with supportive care including intravenous hydration, systemic antibiotics/steroids (e.g., prednisone 80–100 mg/day), and wound care.
- Remove inciting agent or manage infection.
- Use of artificial tears or lubricating ointments (consider tarsorrhaphy if necessary).

- Topical corticosteroid drops (e.g., prednisolone acetate 1% four to eight times per day) and/or antibiotic ointment.
- Topical cycloplegic (e.g., atropine 1% two to four times per day).
- Break symblepharon formation within conjunctival fornices with a glass rod.
- Epilation of lashes if trichiasis develops.
- Consider keratoprosthesis (intracorneal artificial lens) in cases of a very scarred cornea in an eye with visual potential.

■ Follow-up

- Often (daily in acute phase). Monitor corneal involvement and prevent cicatricial changes. Monitor IOP.
- Weekly after acute phase is resolved.
- Monitor for chronic complications.

Acquired Immunodeficiency Syndrome (AIDS)

The prevalence of ophthalmic as well as other systemic comorbidities in AIDS patients increases with the reduction of $CD4^+$ T lymphocytes. In general, once an individual's $CD4^+$ cell population is less than 500 cells/mm^3 the possibility of developing ocular complications becomes more significant. Seventy to eighty percent will be treated for an HIV-associated eye disorder during the course of the illness. Newly available, highly active antiretroviral therapy has lowered the prevalence of ocular complications in patients infected with HIV.

■ History

Disease may range from asymptomatic to symptomatic with blurred vision, floaters, photophobia, pain, and redness—depending on the ocular complications.

■ Clinical Manifestation

Anterior Segment Manifestations

CONJUNCTIVAL NEOPLASMS

- Squamous cell carcinoma
- Kaposi's sarcoma

KAPOSI'S SARCOMA

- Very common in AIDS: 30% of patients; 20% with eyelid or conjunctival involvement (Plate 11)
- May be presenting sign of AIDS although non–vision threatening
- Herpes virus type 8

MOLLUSCUM CONTAGIOSUM

- Most common ocular adnexal manifestation in patients who are HIV positive. The eyelid is involved in 5% of HIV-positive patients.

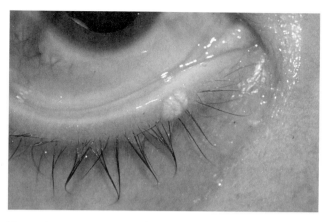

Figure 11-1 • Molluscum lesion with typical umbilicated center.

- DNA pox virus that usually affects children and the elderly.
- Skin nodules around eyes: umbilicated center (Figure 11-1).
- Spreads by direct contact with infected persons.
- Can cause persistent conjunctivitis.

HERPES ZOSTER OPHTHALMICUS
- 5% to 15% of patients who are infected with HIV
- Unusual in young, therefore if present, be suspicious for AIDS
- Can lead to serious eye complications (see Chapter 7, p. 96)

OTHER CONDITIONS
- Infectious keratitis: bacterial, viral (herpetic), fungal (*Candida*), or parasitic (microsporidia)
- Keratoconjunctivitis sicca (dry eye syndrome)
  - More than 20% of AIDS patients have decreased tear production
  - Not related to severity of AIDS
  - May be due to lymphocytic infiltration of lacrimal gland
- Uveitis

Posterior Segment Manifestations

HIV RETINOPATHY
- Most common retinal pathologic process in patients who are HIV positive
- 50% to 70% of patients who are HIV positive
- Cotton-wool spots and occasionally retinal hemorrhages
- Rarely affects vision
- No treatment necessary

CYTOMEGALOVIRUS RETINITIS
- Most common cause of intraocular infection in patients with AIDS

- 40% of patients with advanced HIV infection
- Common in patients with a CD4$^+$ count less than 100 cells/mm^3
- Retinitis: whitening of retina, intraretinal hemorrhages, retina detachment (Plate 24)

OTHER OCULAR INFECTIONS
- Bacterial: syphilis (most common intraocular bacterial infection—2% of HIV positive patients)
- Fungal: cryptococcal chorioretinitis—budding, spore-forming, yeastlike fungus
- Viral: herpetic (progressive outer retinal necrosis)
- Parasitic: *Toxoplasma* chorioretinitis—most common cause of retinochoroiditis.

Neuro-ophthalmic Manifestations
- Numerous abnormalities may occur including: pupillary abnormalities, CN palsies or brain stem ocular motility deficits, optic neuropathy, and visual field defects.
- Etiologies include: CNS infection (e.g., toxoplasmosis), lymphoma, and primary HIV disease.

■ Risk Factors
- Unprotected sexual activity
- Homosexual or bisexual men
- Intravenous drug abuse
- Infants born to HIV-positive mothers
- No antiretroviral treatment when indicated (poor compliance with medications)

■ Treatment
- Kaposi's sarcoma lesions are managed with excision, chemotherapy (e.g., vinblastine and vincristine), and radiation. They often recur but can resolve when patients are given HIV protease inhibitors.
- Molluscum contagiosum is difficult to cure but may be managed with excision or cryotherapy.
- Manage herpes zoster ophthalmicus per Chapter 7.
- Manage uveitis per Chapter 9.
- Treatment for retrobulbar optic neuritis with systemic steroids is absolutely contraindicated in HIV-positive patients until an infectious etiology is ruled out. Systemic steroids further risk immunosuppression and extension of the infection.
- Manage dry eye symptoms with artificial tears, punctal plugs, and cyclosporine emulsion (e.g., Restasis, one drop twice a day).
- Treat cytomegalovirus retinitis with intravenous (e.g., ganciclovir, foscarnet, or cidofovir) or intravitreal (injection or implant) antivirals.

- Associated rhegmatogenous retinal detachments are difficult to manage. May consider "walling off" line of retinitis with laser photocoagulation. Detachments involving the macula are managed with pars plana vitrectomy and silicone oil.

■ Follow-up

- Since the advent of newer, more effective, medication regimens, such as highly active antiretroviral therapy, the proportion of patients developing AIDS-related ocular diseases has greatly decreased. However, ocular disease is still common in this population, and an individual's care should include examination by an ophthalmologist.
- Individuals can be followed as determined by the specific ocular disease.

Sarcoidosis

Common, idiopathic, multisystem, noncaseating granulomatous inflammation most commonly involving pulmonary, neurologic, musculoskeletal, renal, and ocular tissues. Involvement of the eyes and adnexa affects 25% to 54% of patients.

■ Epidemiology

- More common in African Americans and females.
- Overall mortality ranges from 1% to 5%.
- Pulmonary fibrosis and cardiac involvement are the leading causes of death.
- The lungs are affected in about 90% of cases.

■ History

- Neuro-ophthalmologic involvement: symptoms include diplopia from cranial nerve palsies and decreased vision with or without scotoma from optic nerve infiltration or edema.
- Ocular sarcoidosis: uveitis symptoms include blurred vision, photophobia, floaters, redness, scotomata, and pain.
- Periocular and adnexal lesions may produce disfigured lids.
- Orbital involvement may cause proptosis and diplopia.

■ Clinical Manifestation

- Dry eye syndrome due to infiltration of lacrimal glands
- Conjunctival granulomas
- Anterior uveitis (Plate 1): most common ocular manifestation in sarcoidosis
  -Mutton-fat keratic precipitates, iris nodules, posterior synechiae.

- Chronic uveitis can result in cataract, neovascularization (e.g., retina, disc, or iris), glaucoma, and cystoid macular edema (CME).
- Vitritis: snowballs and snowbanking inflammation
- Perivasculitis: limited to retinal veins (candle-wax drippings)
- Choroidal granulomas: multiple, elevated, yellowish nodules

■ Differential Diagnosis

- Tuberculosis: ocular signs are similar to sarcoidosis. Chest radiograph may be abnormal and there may be a positive PPD.
- Idiopathic pars planitis: accumulation of white, fluffy, vitreous opacities and exudates along the pars plana and ora serrata. Debris is usually inferior.
- Includes others causes of uveitis such as infectious, autoimmune, or tumor.

■ Diagnostic Evaluation

- Uveitis workup (see Chapter 9)
- May consider biopsy of conjunctival granulomas, lacrimal gland, lymph node, or skin lesions if present (include acid-fast stain and methenamine-silver stain to rule out TB and fungal infection)
- Angiotensin-converting enzyme (ACE) and lysozyme levels (both may be elevated in sarcoidosis)
- Chest CT or radiograph and pulmonary function tests
- Neuroimaging, lumbar puncture, or electroencephalogram if neurosarcoidosis suspected

■ Treatment

- Anterior uveitis requires aggressive topical steroid treatment (e.g., prednisolone acetate 1%, one drop four to eight times per day) and occasionally oral prednisone (e.g., 30–80 mg PO daily).
- Consider periocular steroid injection (e.g., triamcinolone 20–40 mg) if there is no response to aggressive topical steroids.
- Cycloplegia (e.g., cyclogel 1%, one drop 2–4 times per day) is recommended to relieve ciliary spasm and prevent posterior synechiae formation.
- Manage dry eye with artificial tears, punctal occlusion, and topical cyclosporin A (e.g., Restasis, one drop twice a day). May demonstrate some improvement with oral corticosteroids when dry eye is associated with systemic disease.
- Manage any CME if present with topical steroids or NSAIDs (e.g., ketorolac tromethamine 0.4%, one drop four times per day).

- Manage elevated IOP (caution with prostaglandin analogs-hypotensive lipids if uveitis is present).
- Consider giving systemic steroids or cyclosporin A.
- Cataract surgery if a significant cataract results.

■ Follow-up

- Frequent follow-up as necessary until disease is controlled.
- Children (because of frequent occurrence of asymptomatic uveitis) and patients treated with steroids need more close follow-up.
- Taper steroids as condition improves.
- Monitor IOP carefully if on topical on systemic steroids
- Check serum calcium (to determine if dangerously high levels exist).
- Referral to an internist for a systemic evaluation.

12 Common Ocular Surgery

Thomas E. Bournias, MD and Jerry Lai, MD

Cataract Surgery

Cataracts usually result in slowly progressive visual loss over many months or years. Various symptoms may result, including decreased visual acuity, glare, reduced color perception, and diplopia. There are three major types of cataracts:

1. Nuclear sclerotic: a yellow or brown discoloration of the central portion of the lens. Distance vision is typically affected more than near. This type of cataract usually occurs in individuals older than 60 years.
2. Posterior subcapsular: an opacification, resembling a plaque or sand paper, that forms along the posterior aspect of the lens (Plate 14). Reading difficulty and glare are the most common complaints. It may cause monocular diplopia and is often associated with prolonged use of steroids, ocular inflammation, trauma, diabetes, or exposure to radiation. Posterior subcapsular cataract often occurs in individuals younger than 50 years.
3. Cortical: radial or spokelike opacities that forms in the lens periphery. Cortical cataracts are usually asymptomatic until the spokes develop centrally. The most common symptom is glare.

When the visual symptoms are significant enough to affect a patient's quality of life or ability to function at the desired or necessary level, and corrective contact lenses or glasses do not improve the symptoms, cataract surgery is indicated. Occasionally surgery is performed to correct a narrow angle unresponsive to a laser peripheral iridectomy (LPI) (e.g., phacomorphic glaucoma where a large lens physically narrows the anterior chamber angle) or to facilitate visualization into the back of the eye for subsequent treatment for an underlying condition (e.g., diabetic retinopathy).

The technique for cataract surgery has evolved over the years, requiring progressively smaller incisions and resulting in fewer complications. Techniques include phacoemulsification, extracapsular cataract extraction (ECCE), and intracapsular cataract extraction (ICCE). Today more than 90% of cataract operations

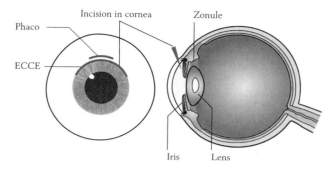

Figure 12-1 • Comparison of 2.5- to 3.0-mm corneal or anterior scleral incision in phacoemulsification with large limbal incision in extracapsular cataract extraction. *(Reprinted with permission from James B, Chew C, Bron A. Lecture notes on ophthalmology, 9th ed. Oxford: Blackwell Publishing Ltd, 2003.)*

are performed by phacoemulsification. ICCE is now very rarely performed. These procedures are briefly discussed below.

■ Phacoemulsification

A 2.5- to 3-mm incision is made through the cornea or sclera (Figure 12-1). After creation of a capsulorrhexis (controlled tear in the anterior lens capsule) to expose the cataractous lens (Figure 12-2), an ultrasound probe is introduced through the incision to remove the cataract in situ by emulsifying (phacoemulsification) the lens (Figure 12-3). The remaining soft lens material (cortex) is then aspirated with another pencil-like instrument (Figure 12-4). An intraocular lens (IOL) is then implanted into

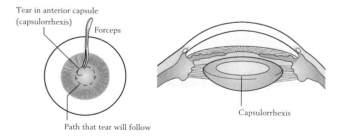

Figure 12-2 • Controlled tear in anterior lens capsule (capsulorrhexis) to expose cataractous lens. *(Reprinted with permission from James B, Chew C, Bron A. Lecture notes on ophthalmology, 9th ed. Oxford: Blackwell Publishing Ltd, 2003.)*

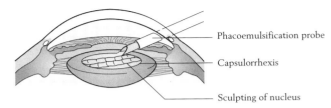

Figure 12-3 • In situ phacoemulsification of the cataract. *(Reprinted with permission from James B, Chew C, Bron A. Lecture notes on ophthalmology, 9th ed. Oxford: Blackwell Publishing Ltd, 2003.)*

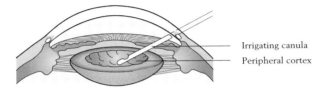

Figure 12-4 • Aspiration of the remaining cortex after phacoemulsification is complete. *(Reprinted with permission from James B, Chew C, Bron A. Lecture notes on ophthalmology, 9th ed. Oxford: Blackwell Publishing Ltd, 2003.)*

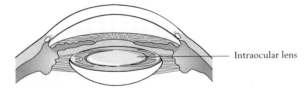

Figure 12-5 • Intraocular lens centered by haptics in the capsular bag. *(Reprinted with permission from James B, Chew C, Bron A. Lecture notes on ophthalmology, 9th ed. Oxford: Blackwell Publishing Ltd, 2003.)*

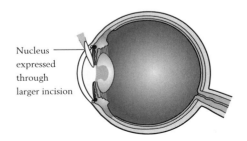

Figure 12-6 • The cataract is expressed en bloc through a larger incision in an extracapsular cataract extraction. *(Reprinted with permission from James B, Chew C, Bron A. Lecture notes on ophthalmology, 9th ed. Oxford: Blackwell Publishing Ltd, 2003.)*

the remaining capsule (capsular bag, Figure 12-5). The wound is then sealed by injection of saline into the edges, resulting in swelling and formation of a watertight wound. This usually results in no need for sutures. However, some surgeons elect to place a single stitch instead.

■ Extracapsular Cataract Extraction

ECCE differs from phacoemulsification in several points: The incision is much larger (Figures 12-1 and 12-2). The nuclear material is expressed en bloc (Figure 12-6) after perforation of the anterior capsule with a ring of small incisions with a needle. The cortex is then aspirated, and an IOL is placed in the capsular bag as in phacoemulsification. Several sutures are required to close the larger incision.

■ Intracapsular Cataract Extraction

ICCE is rarely performed but is necessary when the zonules (fibers from lens equator to the ciliary body) that support the lens are weakened and incapable of safely allowing surgical manipulation of the lens. A large incision, as in an ECCE, near the limbus is created. The lens with its intact capsular bag is grasped with an erisiphake (suction cup) or cryoprobe (metal-tipped probe with temperature reduced to freezing) and removed en bloc with the surrounding capsule. Since there is no resultant capsular support, the IOL is placed in the anterior chamber (AC). This procedure results in a higher rate of complications.

■ Complications

Opacification of the posterior capsule occurs weeks to years later in 20% to 30% of patients. It may be managed in the office with a neodymium: yttrium-aluminum-garnet (Nd:YAG) laser that cuts the opacified capsule open (capsulotomy). This procedure is associated with a slightly higher risk of retinal detachment. See Box 12-1 for additional complications.

■ Postoperative Management

In small incisional surgery, postoperative recovery is quick. Usually patients use topical antibiotics for 3 to 7 days and topical steroids (e.g., prednisolone acetate 1%, one drop four times per day or loteprednol etabonate 0.5%, one drop four times per day) or non-steroidal anti-inflammatory drugs (e.g., ketorolac tromethamine 0.4%, one drop four times per day) for 1 to 2 weeks. A new glasses prescription (if necessary) is given in 1 to 3 weeks. A dilated

■ **BOX 12-1 Complications of Cataract Surgery**

Endophthalmitis
Retinal detachment
Corneal edema
Cystoid macular edema (edematous macula)
Retained lens fragments
Vitreous loss
Glaucoma
Iris prolapse in the wound
Wound distortion or disruption
Astigmatism (e.g., from tight sutures)
Flat or shallow anterior chamber from wound leak
Hemorrhage
Intraocular lens dislocation
Opacified posterior capsule

fundus examination is performed during the postoperative period to assure that no retinal hole or detachment has developed (especially if intraoperative posterior capsular rupture or vitreous loss occurred).

Glaucoma Surgery

Patients with glaucoma who demonstrate progression of disease or inadequate IOP despite maximally tolerated medical therapy with or without previous laser trabeculoplasty or those who are not compliant with, or cannot afford, medications are candidates for glaucoma filtration surgery. Guarded filtration surgery, or trabeculectomy, is the most widely used incisional glaucoma procedure.

■ Trabeculectomy

The goal of a trabeculectomy (Figure 12-7) is to create a fistula between the AC and subconjunctival space. It usually results in substantial reduction in IOP and has increasingly been used earlier in the management of uncontrolled glaucoma. An incision is created in the conjunctive in the fornix or at the limbus and is dissected and reflected exposing the underlying scleral bed. A partial thickness scleral flap is created and dissection is carried to clear cornea. At this point the eye is entered with a surgical blade and a small opening (sclerostomy) is made by excising TM and sclera. A small section of the iris is excised in this area (iridectomy) to prevent blockage of the sclerostomy. This allows egress

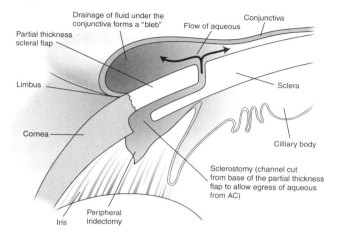

Figure 12-7 • Schematic demonstrating a section through a trabeculectomy. A fistula is created to allow egress of aqueous from the anterior chamber to the subconjunctival space to lower the IOP. Suturing the overlying partial thickness scleral flap over the fistula helps regulate the amount of egressing aqueous and thereby controlling the IOP.

of aqueous from the AC to the subconjunctival space. Numerous sutures are placed through the scleral flap to control the flow of the egressing aqueous. The conjunctiva is then sutured in a water-tight fashion with subsequent formation of a "bleb" (Figure 12-8).

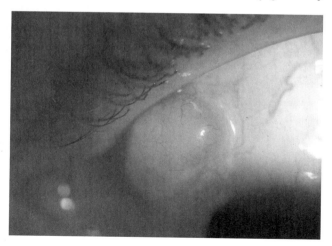

Figure 12-8 • "Bleb."

From here, the aqueous apparently drains into the conjunctival vasculature resulting in lower IOP. Antifibrotic agents, such as mitomycin-C (0.2–0.5 mg/cc for 2 to 5 minutes) and 5-fluorouracil (50 mg/mL for 2 to 5 minutes), are often used at the time of surgery to decrease postoperative fibrosis and subsequent failure of the bleb. On occasion, postoperative subconjunctival 5-FU (5 mg/0.1 cc) injections are given. Common complications are outlined in Box 12-2.

■ Postoperative Management

Topical antibiotics, cycloplegics (to deepen the AC) (e.g., atropine 1%, one drop two to four times per day), and steroids (e.g., prednisolone acetate 1%, one drop four to eight times per day) (to reduce inflammation and subsequent scarring) are used. Topical steroids are often used for 6 to 12 weeks. The postoperative management is rarely uneventful, often necessitating the use of subconjunctival 5-FU injections (to slow scarring/healing) or laser suture lysis (or removal of releasable sutures) to increase flow of aqueous to the subconjunctival space. Postoperative complications such as hypotony (low IOP, less than 6 mm Hg) and a shallow AC are common.

■ BOX 12-2 Complications of Filtration Surgery

Early Complications
Bleb leak
Flat anterior chamber (from bleb leak or overfiltration)
Hypotony (from bleb leak or overfiltration)
Hyphema
Infection/endophthalmitis
Transient IOP elevation
Formation/acceleration of cataract
Choroidal effusion/hemorrhage

Late Complications
Bleb leakage
Failure (scarring) of bleb
Cataract formation
Infection/blebitis/endophthalmitis
Symptomatic bleb (i.e., pain)
Hypotony
Hypotony maculopathy

■ Other Glaucoma Procedures

Aqueous Shunt (Setons)

An aqueous drainage device, such as the Baerveldt, Ahmed, or Molteno, is often used after two or more previously failed trabeculectomies, if there is excessive conjunctival scarring that precludes trabeculectomy, or in neovascular glaucoma. In this procedure, a plate is sutured into the subconjunctival space. A connected tube is placed in the AC through the limbus or in the posterior portion of the eye through the pars plana. The aqueous from the AC (or posterior portion of the eye) then flows through the tube to the plate. Excellent reductions in IOP may be obtained but with an increased incidence of complications, especially hypotony.

Deep Sclerectomy (Nonpenetrating Filtration Surgery)

A procedure similar to trabeculectomy but the AC is not entered. Entry is made into Schlemm's canal but Descemet's membrane is not removed. There is a lower incidence of postoperative hypotony, but long-term results are controversial.

Cyclodestructive Procedures

Performed in glaucoma patients who do not respond to conventional incisional glaucoma surgery, have uveitic or neovascular glaucoma, or have a blind eye but are experiencing pain. A cryoprobe (freezing probe) or laser (e.g., diode) is applied near the limbus with resulting destruction of the underlying ciliary processes of the ciliary body. This usually results in less aqueous production and lower IOP. Diode laser is associated with less pain, inflammation, and hypotony than cryotherapy.

Laser Peripheral Iridectomy

LPI is usually performed in eyes with a narrow or closed angle (angle-closure glaucoma). A thermal laser (e.g., argon) or, most commonly, a "cutting" laser (i.e., Nd:YAG) creates a tiny hole in the peripheral iris to allow egress of aqueous from the posterior chamber to the AC, thus relieving the pupillary block. The peripheral iris then falls back relieving obstruction of the TM.

Laser Trabeculoplasty

Argon Laser Trabeculoplasty

Argon laser trabeculoplasty (ALT) is performed in patients with open angles who may or may not be currently taking glaucoma medications. Using a gonioscopy lens, 50 to 100 applications of a thermal laser are applied to the trabecular meshwork (TM) over 180 to 360 degrees resulting in lower IOP in about two thirds of patients. Patients with pigment dispersion syndrome (PDS) or pseudoexfoliation (PXE) have a higher success rate of significant IOP reduction of about 90%. Generally, repeating this procedure after having previously treated 360 degrees of trabecular meshwork provides no further benefit.

SELECTIVE LASER TRABECULOPLASTY

Similar to ALT but with minimal to no thermal effect on the TM. Selective laser trabeculoplasty (SLT) may be repeated after previous ALT or SLT. Long-term data regarding efficacy are limited.

Corneal Refractive Surgery

The refractive state of the eye is determined by corneal power, AC depth, lens power, and axial length. Since the cornea accounts for two thirds of the refractive power of the eye, alterations in its shape may result in dramatic changes for an eye's refractive error. Individuals with significant myopia, hyperopia, or astigmatism are increasingly undergoing these procedures to reduce or eliminate the need for spectacle correction. Other indications for corneal refractive surgery are intolerance to contact lenses or glasses, or to improve induced refractive error from previous ocular surgery. Persons who are presbyopic (older than 40 years) will still need reading glasses to varying degrees. The procedure most commonly performed today is laser-assisted in situ keratomileusis (LASIK). Some patients undergo photorefractive keratectomy (PRK) and very rarely now radial keratotomy (RK) with or without astigmatic keratotomy (AK). A new technique (called conductive keratoplasty or CK) to improve presbyopia (loss of near or accomodative vision) has just been approved by the FDA.

■ Laser-Assisted In Situ Keratomileusis (LASIK)

Generally performed on eyes with 0.5 to 12.0 diopters of myopia, 0.5 to 4.0 diopters of hyperopia, and up to 8.0 diopters of astigmatism. This procedure is performed in eyes that have sufficient corneal thickness. Pneumatic suction is applied to the cornea (increasing the IOP of the eye) so that a microkeratome creates a uniform 160-µm thick corneal flap. Thinner flaps may be created by a fematosecond laser. The flap is lifted and an ultraviolet laser (193-nm excimer) ablates midstromal corneal tissue to modify its curvature. The flap is then irrigated and repositioned.

■ Photorefractive Keratectomy

Generally performed on eyes with up to 8.0 diopters of myopia and mild to moderate hyperopia and/or astigmatism. It is also performed to treat superficial corneal scars or basement membrane changes resulting in recurrent corneal erosion. In this technique, the epithelium is removed from the cornea and the excimer laser ablates Bowman's layer and the superficial corneal stroma to modify the corneal curvature. A bandage contact lens is placed over the cornea to allow the epithelium to heal (usually over 1 to 3 days). This procedure is associated with more pain because of the large epithelial defect.

■ Radial Keratotomy

Rarely performed now but generally can be performed on eyes with up to 5.0 diopters of myopia (does not correct hyperopia). In this procedure, a series of deep, radial, corneal stromal incisions are made (from a 4–6 mm optical zone to the limbus) with a diamond blade through 90% to 95% of the corneal thickness. This causes weakening of the paracentral and peripheral cornea, resulting in flattening of the surface. Astigmatism may also be corrected by arcuate (parallel to the limbus) or tangential incisions (termed astigmatic keratotomy or AK) that flatten the cornea along the incisional meridian. LASIK and PRK involve ablation of central corneal tissue, but RK avoids the central corneal tissue. However, RK and AK weaken corneal integrity and result in a higher risk for a ruptured globe after trauma.

■ Contraindications/Cautions (for corneal refractive surgery)

- Severe dry eyes
- History of herpetic corneal disease
- Corneal ectasias (or thinning such as keratoconus)
- Uveitis
- Progressive retinal disease
- Large pupil size
- Thin cornea (with LASIK) as measured by pachymetry
- Poor wound healing such as in diabetes
- Complications for these procedures are outlined in Table 12-1.

■ TABLE 12-1 Complications of Corneal Refractive Surgery

Procedure	Complications
All	Glare, halos
	Undercorrection/overcorrection
	Regression/progression of refractive error
	Infectious keratitis/infiltrate
	Complication of topical steroids (e.g., stromal melt, infectious keratitis)
	Worsening of dry eye
	Steroid-induced glaucoma
PRK	Pain
	Corneal haze or scar formation
	Recurrent erosion syndrome
LASIK	Flap complications (lost, thin, folds, button-hole)
	Epithelium ingrowth
	"Sands of Sahara"
	Keratectasia
	Corneal haze
	Intraocular penetration (also with RK/AK)

Note: Decrease in corneal thickness results in overestimation of corneal power by keratometers (used for intraocular lens selection for cataract surgery) as well as underestimation of IOP by applanation tonometry.

A Opportunities in Ophthalmology

Ophthalmology residency focuses on the prevention, diagnosis, and management of disease and abnormalities of the eye and periocular structures. An excellent combination of office-based clinical medicine and outpatient surgery is provided. A one-year transitional year or internship in medicine, surgery, pediatrics, or neurology prior to beginning residency is required. Most ophthalmology residency training programs are 3 years in duration.

Many residency programs emphasize high class rank and research experience for applicants. Ophthalmology has a reputation as being "difficult to enter," but it has become easier to gain acceptance over the last decade. Ophthalmology remains a popular and competitive specialty for medical students. Approximately half of all graduating ophthalmology residents enter subspecialty fellowships, including glaucoma, cornea and external disease, refractive surgery, retina, neuro-ophthalmology, oculoplastics, pediatric ophthalmology, uveitis, and pathology.

For further information, contact the Ophthalmology Residency Matching Program (OMP), P.O. Box 7584, San Francisco, CA 94120-7584, www.sfmatch.org.

The Central Application Service (CAS) will distribute your applications to each program requested. Applications should be returned to CAS by late August (2 years prior to beginning residency). Five to eight interviews are generally recommended to increase the likelihood of acceptance. Rank order lists are submitted by mid-January with announcement of selected applications later that month. Match results are obtained before the National Resident Matching Program (NRMP) rank order lists.

Recent statistics for applicants:

Number of ACGME-approved programs	122
Number of entry level spots for matriculation (in 2003)	452
Percent of matriculated residents female	32
Number of applications in 2002	671
Percent of matriculating residency foreign graduates	7.9
Average USMLE score for all matriculated	225
Average resident hours per week	49

B Review Questions and Answers

QUESTIONS

1. A neurologically normal, obese 24-year-old woman loses vision whenever she stands up suddenly. She is uncertain whether one or both eyes are involved, but is sure that involvement is never longer than 1 minute. Which of the following is most likely?

   A. Arnold-Chiari malformation
   B. Increased intracranial pressure
   C. Ischemic optic neuropathy
   D. Ocular transient ischemic attack
   E. Teratoma of the hypothalamus

2. Axons of retinal ganglion cells travel through the optic nerve and pass through the optic foramen to the optic chiasma where they partially decussate. Mixed fibers from the two optic nerves continue through the optic tracts and end in the following structure:

   A. Caudate nucleus
   B. Ciliary ganglion
   C. Edinger-Westphal nucleus
   D. Lateral geniculate body
   E. Pterygopalatine ganglion

3. Which of the following regarding leukocoria is true?

   A. It is always associated with a media opacity.
   B. It is often associated with aniridia.
   C. It is usually bilateral
   D. It may be associated with persistent hyperplastic primary vitreous.
   E. It rarely results in amblyopia

4. An 80-year-old woman presents to the emergency room with abrupt painless loss of vision in the right eye. Her only other symptoms are temporal headache and some pain when chewing food. Upon examination, she is found to have a pale fundus, narrowed arterioles, and a cherry-red spot in the right eye. What is the most important next step in evaluation?

   A. Cardiac echocardiogram
   B. Carotid ultrasound
   C. Erythrocyte sedimentation rate

D. Fluorescein angiography

E. Hypercoagulability panel

5. The funduscopic examination in ophthalmic artery occlusion differs from that of central artery occlusion in which of the following ways?

A. A cherry-red spot usually occurs only in central retinal artery occlusion (CRAO).

B. A choroidal neovascular membrane is seen only in ophthalmic artery occlusion.

C. Hypertension is a risk for CRAO but not for ophthalmic artery occlusion.

D. Ischemic whitening of the retina only occurs in ophthalmic artery occlusion.

E. There is good definitive therapy only for ophthalmic artery occlusion.

6. Recent research has shown regular supplementation with which of the following to be preventative in the development of age-related macular degeneration?

A. Calcium

B. Ginseng

C. Magnesium

D. Selenium

E. Zinc

7. A 60-year-old woman presents to her ophthalmologist complaining of blurry vision and distortion of objects. Upon examination, she is found to perceive blurry lines on Amsler grid testing, as well as to have chorioretinal atrophy, multiple drusen, and pigment irregularities on funduscopic examination. Which of the following would most likely put her at risk for also having a choroidal neovascular membrane in the future?

A. Age greater than 65 years

B. Drusen greater than 64 μm

C. Hypertension

D. Microaneurysms

E. Smoking more than two packs per day

8. Which of the following is true regarding herpes zoster ophthalmicus (HZO)?

A. It is a reactivation of latent varicella-zoster virus laying dormant in the facial nerve.

B. It may cause uveitis, in which case topical steroids are indicated.

C. It may develop increased corneal sensitivity.

D. Most patients are 20 to 30 years old.

E. The treatment of choice is topical antiviral medication.

9. A patient presents with reduced visual acuity and pain in her left eye. Upon examination, one third of the anterior chamber is filled with blood. She has no history of ocular surgery but recently was

involved in a sports-related injury to her eye. She did not think it was serious and so sought no medical attention until the pain became worse. What examination finding is most likely expected?

A. Corneal ulceration
B. Foreign body sensation
C. Positive Seidel test result
D. Relative afferent pupillary defect
E. Staining of the cornea

10. A 42-year-old woman arrives in the emergency room 2 hours after a car accident. When she crashed into another vehicle, the airbag opened and struck her on the face. At the time of presentation she complained of sharp pain in her left eye associated with tearing and sensitivity to light. Upon slit lamp examination, the iris looked displaced. Intraocular pressure is low in the traumatized eye. The rest of the eye examination would more likely show:

A. Cup/disc asymmetry
B. Detachment of the retina
C. Kayser-Fleischer ring
D. Roth's spots
E. White blood cells and flare in the anterior chamber

11. Which of the following is true in testing the pupils?

A. A relative afferent pupillary defect occurs when one sees a stronger consensual reflex than direct reflex.
B. The consensual reflex is when the pupil constricts in the illuminated eye.
C. The direct reflex is when the pupil constricts in the nonilluminated eye.
D. The pupils cannot be tested directly.
E. The swinging flashlight test does not compare the consensual and direct reflexes.

12. Upon testing the visual acuity for a 68-year-old man, the fourth-year medical student found the patient's vision to be 20/100. With the use of the pinhole test, the vision did not change. Which of the following is most likely to account for this poor vision?

A. Hyperopia
B. Hyperopia with mild astigmatism
C. Incorrect prescription for his glasses
D. Myopia with mild astigmatism
E. Nuclear cataract

13. A patient was told that he had macular degeneration. His visual acuity was 20/50 in both eyes. The test that can be used to assess macular function is:

A. Amsler grid test
B. Anterior chamber examination
C. A-scan ultrasonography

D. Fluorescein angiography

E. Frequency-doubling technology perimetry

14. A 63-year-old Hispanic woman was referred to the specialized clinic because she had recently developed uveitis. The patient asked the doctor about the meaning of uveitis. The doctor answered that it is an inflammation of the part of the eye called the uvea. The uvea is composed of the following structures:

    A. Choroid, retina, iris

    B. Choroid, retinal pigment epithelium, ciliary body

    C. Iris, choroid, and ciliary body

    D. Iris, ciliary body, retinal pigment epithelium

    E. Retina, ciliary body, lens

15. A 35-year-old woman recently diagnosed with thyroid eye disease has clinically apparent lid retraction, 2 mm of proptosis bilaterally, and symptoms of dry eyes. Her vision is 20/20 without limitations in motility or color vision; however, she has 1 mm of lagophthalmos in both eyes. The best course of treatment for this patient includes:

    A. Artificial tears and ointment at night

    B. Better control of thyroid function to decrease the proptosis

    C. Eyelid closing procedure to limit exposure (lateral tarsorrhaphy)

    D. Orbital decompression surgery to reduce proptosis

    E. Radiation therapy to minimize orbital involvement

16. Which of the following regarding glaucoma is true?

    A. All patients with an intraocular pressure (IOP) greater than 21 mm Hg should be treated until the IOP is 20 mm Hg or less.

    B. Central corneal thickness measurements by pachymetry help to determine the overall risk of glaucoma patients.

    C. First-line management of uveitic glaucoma should always be with prostaglandin analog-hypotensive lipid drops.

    D. It is always associated with elevated IOP (greater than 21 mm Hg).

    E. Peripheral visual field test results may be normal.

17. The action of pilocarpine at the iris sphincter muscle is analogous to the action of what drug at the iris dilator muscle?

    A. Atropine

    B. Cocaine

    C. Epinephrine

    D. Hydroxyamphetamine (Parderine)

    E. Timolol

18. Which of the following is true when trying to differentiate episcleritis from scleritis?

    A. Episcleritis only occurs in one eye, whereas scleritis typically occurs in both eyes.

    B. The inflamed vessels in episcleritis blanch with topical phenylephrine.

  C. The inflamed vessels in episcleritis cannot be moved with a cotton-tipped applicator.

  D. The vessels form a criss-cross pattern in episcleritis as opposed to a radial pattern in scleritis.

  E. The vessels in episcleritis are violet-blue, as opposed to bright red in scleritis.

19. Which of the following is true regarding pingueculae?

  A. If left unmanaged, they will always develop into pterygia.

  B. If not excised, will always cause pain and irritation.

  C. They are located on the cornea.

  D. They may interfere with contact lens wear.

  E. They are rarely bilateral.

20. The most common posterior segment manifestation in patients with AIDS is:

  A. Cytomegalovirus retinitis

  B. HIV retinopathy

  C. Optic neuritis

  D. Retinal detachment

  E. *Toxoplasma* chorioretinitis

21. A 32-year-old woman presents with sudden onset of right eye pain and blurry vision. She states that she is very photophobic and has noted some thick discharge from the affected eye. The patient has no past medical history. The only ocular history the patient provides is that she has worn contact lenses for many years and occasionally sleeps with her lenses still in. Which of the following findings will most likely be found on examination?

  A. A scleral nodule that is immobile and deep red-purple

  B. Corneal epithelial defect with underlying dense white stromal inflammation with indistinct edges

  C. Dendritic corneal epithelial ulcer

  D. Thinning of the inferior paracentral cornea, with scissoring of the red reflex on retinoscopy

  E. Wing-shaped fold of conjunctiva and fibrovascular tissue that has invaded the superficial cornea

22. Recurrent erosions:

  A. Always result from previous ocular trauma and/or corneal abrasions

  B. Are typically treated with topical steroids

  C. Can only be diagnosed when a frank corneal epithelial defect is found

  D. May be managed with epithelial debridement

  E. Occur due to poor adhesion of the corneal endothelium to Descemet's membrane

23. The eye movement is coordinated by four recti and two oblique muscles. The only extraocular muscle that does not originate from the orbital apex is:

    A. Inferior rectus
    B. Inferior oblique
    C. Lateral rectus
    D. Superior oblique
    E. Superior rectus

24. A 55-year-old African-American man presents to the clinic with a history of glaucoma. The fourth-year medical student explains to him that the aqueous humor produced by the ciliary processes drains out mainly through the conventional pathway. However, the nonconventional pathway accounts for about 10% of aqueous outflow. The patient asks where the nonconventional pathway is. The answer should be:

    A. Schlemm's canal
    B. The 25 to 30 collector channels
    C. Trabecular meshwork
    D. Uveoscleral outflow
    E. Zonules

25. Which of the following is most likely to be associated with a retinal tear in a phakic eye?

    A. History of blunt trauma
    B. Light flashes
    C. Moderate anterior segment cells and flare
    D. Pigmented granules in the vitreous
    E. Vitreous hemorrhage

ANSWER KEY

1. B	10. E	19. D
2. D	11. A	20. B
3. D	12. E	21. B
4. C	13. A	22. D
5. A	14. C	23. B
6. E	15. A	24. D
7. B	16. E	25. D
8. B	17. C	
9. E	18. B	

ANSWERS

1. **B. The patient's sex, obesity, lack of other neurologic symptoms, and the character of visual loss all suggest that these episodes are the "transient obscurations of vision" associated with chronically elevated intracranial pressure, most likely due to pseudotumor cerebri. When she stands up, the perfusion pressure to the optic nerve drops transiently.** Transient ischemic attacks are usually monocular and of longer duration. They usually involve individuals who are older in the atherosclerotic age range. Clinically, orthostatic hypertension may be included in the differential diagnosis.

2. **D. Visual fibers passing through the optic tracts synapse in the lateral geniculate body and ultimately end in the cortex of the occipital lobe in the brain.** The ciliary ganglion contains parasympathetic efferent fibers. Parasympathetic afferent fibers synapse in the Edinger-Westphal nucleus located in the midbrain.

3. **D. Leukocoria may be seen in congenitally cloudy corneas, cataracts, persistent hyperplastic primary vitreous, uveitis, retinopathy of prematurity (ROP), retinoblastoma, Coat's disease, and toxocariasis.** It is typically unilateral and often may result in amblyopia, even if treated. It is not always associated with media opacity—especially if it is secondary to retinal disorders such as ROP ands retinoblastoma. Aniridia is typically not associated with leukocoria.

4. **C. One must rule out temporal arteritis in all patients older than 50 years with sudden loss of vision or a central retinal artery occlusion (CRAO) with an ESR measurement.** Since this patient has suggestive symptoms of headache and jaw claudication, it would be prudent to also start corticosteroids immediately as this can help decrease the incidence of CRAO in the fellow eye. Once it is determined that the patient does not have temporal arteritis, the other tests may be done to look for other causes of her CRAO.

5. **A.** Hypertension is a risk factor for both conditions, and there is no proven therapy for either. Ischemic whitening of the retina occurs in both, while **there is usually no cherry-red spot in ophthalmic artery occlusion.** A choroidal neovascular membrane is not a feature of either condition.

6. **E. Recent research shows regular use of zinc and antioxidants may be preventative in the development of age-related macular degeneration.** There are no data supporting definite benefit of any of the other nutrients.

7. **B. Drusen greater than 64 μm in size and focal retinal pigment epithelium hyperpigmentation place a patient at high risk for subsequent choroidal neovascular membrane development.** The other choices are risk factors for developing age-related macular degeneration, but not necessarily for neovascular membrane development.

8. **B. Herpes zoster ophthalmicus (HZO) can cause inflammation of almost any ocular tissue, including cornea, uveal tissue, episclera, sclera, choroid, retina, and optic nerve. In addition to systemic antiviral medication, such as acyclovir, a topical steroid is indicated for uveitis.** Topical antivirals are not effective against HZO. HZO represents a reactivation of latent varicella-zoster virus laying dormant in the ophthalmic division of the trigeminal nerve, not the facial nerve. Most patients are 60 to 90 years old, and many are on immunosuppressive therapy. Diminished corneal sensation develops in 50% of patients with HZO.

9. **E. This patient presents with a traumatic hyphema, which is associated with corneal staining due to the prolonged presence of blood in the anterior chamber.** Photophobia and foreign body sensation are more consistent with corneal abrasion. A positive Seidel test result is usually seen with a corneal foreign body and a perforating wound. Corneal ulceration would not present with blood in the anterior chamber.

10. **E. As a result of trauma, the patient developed inflammation of the iris, or traumatic iritis, characterized by anterior chamber reaction (white blood cells and flare).** Roth's spots are hemorrhages with white centers seen in conditions such as leukemia and collagen vascular diseases, but not as a result of trauma. Patients with retinal detachment usually complain of flashes of light in their vision, although retinal detachment could occur after trauma. Cup/disc asymmetry is a sign of glaucoma and does not develop directly after trauma. A Kayser-Fleischer ring is seen in Wilson's disease due to accumulation of copper in the corneal periphery and not as a result of trauma.

11. **A.** The direct reflex is defined as pupil constriction in the illuminated eye. The consensual reflex is defined as pupil constriction in the nonilluminated eye. The swinging flashlight test *does* compare the

consensual and direct reflexes by alternately shining brisk light on each eye and observing pupillary response. **It is true that a relative afferent pupillary defect occurs when one sees a stronger consensual reflex than direct reflex.**

12. **E.** The pinhole test only allows central rays of light into the eye, so that the patient does not need to use their refractive surfaces to view images. Since the visual acuity did not improve with the pinhole test, refractive error is less likely to be the cause of poor vision. **A nuclear cataract could account for no visual acuity improvement with the pinhole test.**

13. **A. The Amsler grid test is used to assess macular function. It tests the central 10 to 20 degrees of the visual field in each eye.** Fluorescein angiography is used to study blood circulation of the retina and the underlying choroid and does not directly test macular function. Frequency-doubling technology (FDT) perimetry is a test of the visual fields. An A-scan ultrasonographic examination is used to make axial length measurements and to examine structures in the eye that are not visible. This test does not assess macular function. Anterior chamber examination is performed to study structures in the anterior portion of the eye. The macula is located in the posterior pole of the eye.

14. **C. The uvea is composed of three structures: iris, choroid, and ciliary body.** The other answers are incorrect.

15. **A. This patient only has symptoms of dry eyes and exposure at night, which can be managed adequately with artificial tears, lubricating ointment, and punctal plugs.** This patient does not have any of the signs of optic nerve compression or ocular motility issues, and orbital decompression or strabismus surgery is not needed. Eyelid surgery is reserved in severe cases. It should not be done prior to decompression and muscle surgery if needed. Management of hyper- or hypothyroid state does not reverse the chronic changes that occur within the extraocular muscles. Occasionally, acute exacerbations of ocular symptoms resolve, but not secondary to better control of thyroid function.

16. **E.** The normal range for intraocular pressure (IOP) is 10 to 21 mm Hg. About 30% to 40% of glaucoma patients are never found to have an elevated IOP greater than 21 mm Hg (normal-tension glaucoma). The majority of patients with elevated IOP (more than 21 mm Hg) do not have glaucoma (ocular hypertensives); therefore, not all patients with elevated IOP need to be treated. Prostaglandin analog-hypotensive lipids have been implicated to exacerbate or cause inflammation and therefore should be used cautiously in uveitic eyes. Central corneal thickness by pachymetry has been found to predict relative risk in ocular hypertensives without glaucoma; there are very few prospective data in patients with actual glaucoma. **Early glaucoma is defined as a characteristic optic**

nerve cupping **without the presence of visual field defects on automated visual fields.**

17. **C. Epinephrine, like pilocarpine, directly stimulates muscle receptor sites.** Atropine blocks sphincter muscle receptors and prevents stimulation by cholinergic drugs, indirectly producing pupillary dilation (mydriasis). Cocaine blocks re-uptake of norepinephrine at the presynaptic terminal at the pupillary dilator muscle, thereby promoting dilation indirectly. Hydroxyamphetamine (Paradrine) releases norepinephrine from the presynaptic terminal, but does not directly act at the pupillary dilator muscle receptors. Timolol is a glaucoma drug (beta blocker) which inhibits production of aqueous at the ciliary body.

18. **B. One of the key diagnostic tests to distinguish episcleritis from scleritis is that the inflamed vessels in episcleritis blanch with topical phenylephrine.** The two diseases can also be differentiated by localizing the site of inflammation to the episclera, in which the inflamed vessels of episcleritis can be moved with a cotton-tipped applicator. The vessels in episcleritis are bright red and form a radial pattern, whereas those in scleritis are violet-blue and form a criss-cross pattern. Both diseases may affect both eyes from one third to one half of the time.

19. **D. The indications for excision of pingueculae include interference with successful contact lens wear, chronic inflammation with redness or pain, and cosmesis.** Though pterygia are almost always preceded and accompanied by pingueculae, not all pinguecule develop into pterygia. Bouts of recurrent inflammation and ocular irritation may be encountered with pingueculae, but only in some cases. Pingueculae are usually bilateral. They usually occur on the nasal and temporal anterior bulbar conjunctiva near the limbus.

20. **B. The most common posterior segment manifestation in patients with AIDS is HIV retinopathy.** Cytomegalovirus retinitis is the most common posterior segment *infection* in patients with AIDS. The others are not common posterior segment findings in patients with AIDS.

21. **B. Given the history of contact lens overuse and symptoms of acute eye pain, blurry vision, and mucopurulent discharge, this patient most likely has an infectious corneal ulcer. The findings in choice (b) are consistent with a bacterial infection; patients who wear their contact lenses overnight have a 15-fold greater risk of infection.** The findings in choice (a) are consistent with nodular anterior scleritis, which has more of a gradual onset and no mucopurulent discharge. The findings in choice (c) are consistent with herpes simplex virus keratitis, which may present in a similar manner as above; however, given that the patient admits to contact lens overuse and is not immunocompromised, this is less likely. The findings in choice (d) are consistent with keratoconus, which may cause blurry

vision but typically no pain (unless the patient develops acute hydrops), photophobia, or discharge. The findings in choice (e) are consistent with pterygium, which may cause blurry vision and irritation, but no discharge or photophobia.

22. **D. Recurrent erosions have a variety of treatment options, including (1) frequent lubrication, antibiotic ointments and cycloplegia, followed by hypertonic saline solutions; (2) therapeutic contact lens with concomitant use of topical antibiotic; (3) anterior stromal micropuncture, (4) epithelial debridement, and (5) excimer laser phototherapeutic keratectomy. The goal for all of these treatments is to promote proper epithelial attachment to its underlying basement membrane.** Topical steroids are not used to manage recurrent erosions. Recurrent erosions occur due to poor adhesion of the corneal epithelium to its underlying basement membrane. Many patients seem to suffer from ocular discomfort out of proportion to the amount of observable pathology; sometimes only subtle corneal abnormalities can be found, and a frank epithelial defect is not necessary for diagnosis. Recurrent erosions may result from previous ocular trauma/corneal abrasion, as well as from preexisting epithelial basement membrane dystrophy.

23. **B. The inferior oblique muscle is the only muscle that does not originate from the apex of the orbit. It originates from the orbital floor nasally, near the orbital rim.** The rest of the above-mentioned muscles originate from the orbital apex.

24. **D. Fluid in the nonconventional pathway drains across the ciliary body into the supraciliary space. This is called the uveoscleral outflow.** The conventional pathway goes through the trabecular meshwork, Schlemm's canal, and thereafter through 25 to 30 collector channels. The zonules are the supporting attachments of the lens to the spaces between the ciliary processes.

25. **D. Pigmented granules (Shafer's sign) are almost pathognomonic of a retinal tear or retinal detachment in an eye that has never had intraocular surgery.** All of the others may be seen in eyes with retinal tears or retinal detachments; but many patients may have these signs and symptoms without having a tear or detachment.

C Common Ophthalmic Medications

Drug packaging standards have generally been adopted for topical medications to help reduce confusion in labeling and identification. The standard colors for drug labels or bottle caps are listed in Table C-1.

■ **TABLE C-1 Topical Ophthalmic Drug Packing Standards**

Therapeutic Class	Color
Beta blockers	Yellow, blue, or both
Mydriatics and cycloplegics	Red
Adrenergics	Purple
Miotics	Green
NSAIDs	Gray
Anti-infective agents	Brown, tan
Carbonic anhydrase inhibitors	Orange
Prostaglandin analogues/hypotensive lipids	Teal

Note: The following list of medications includes many of the most commonly used drugs in ophthalmologic practice. Indications and mechanisms of action as well as common contraindications, cautions, and side effects are listed. *Additional cautions and contraindications* for most of these drugs include allergy to the drug or any of its components, significant hepatic or renal disease, use in infants as well as in pregnant or breast-feeding women.

Acetazolamide (e.g., Diamox, 250 mg PO four times per day or Diamox Sequel 500 mg PO two times per day)

   Indication: elevated IOP, benign intracranial hypertension (pseudotumor cerebri)

   Mechanism: carbonic anhydrase inhibitor (decreased aqueous production)

   Contraindication: sulfa allergy, metabolic acidosis, adrenal insufficiency

   Caution: history of kidney stones, concurrent use of another diuretic, systemic steroid, digoxin (acetazolamide may lower serum potassium significantly)

Side effects: kidney stones, blood dyscrasias, tingling in extremities, taste perversion

Apraclonidine (e.g., Iopidine 0.5%–1.0%; topical, two to three times per day)

Indication: elevated intraocular pressure (IOP), premedication for laser eye surgery

Mechanism: α-receptor agonist, primarily α_1 (decreased aqueous production)

Contraindication: concurrent use of monoamine oxidase inhibitors

Side effects: ocular: allergy, lid retraction, mydriasis (pupil dilation); systemic: dizziness, fatigue, dry mouth

Atropine (topical)

Indication: pupillary dilation (mydriasis), inhibiting accommodation (cycloplegia); for refracting pediatric patients or managing strabismus; deepen the anterior chamber (postoperative, e.g., after glaucoma surgery)

Mechanism: cholinergic antagonist to receptors at pupillary sphincter (mydriasis) and ciliary body (cycloplegia)

Contraindication: angle closure, albinos, infants, Down syndrome

Caution: pediatric patients (toxicity)

Side effects: urinary retention, tachycardia, delirium

Note: recovery: 7 to 10 days

Bimatoprost (e.g., Lumigan; topical, once at night)

Indication: elevated IOP

Mechanism: primary: increased outflow facility, secondary: increased uveoscleral outflow (prostaglandin analog-hypotensive lipid, Prostamide)

Contraindication: cystoid macular edema, history of herpetic corneal disease, pregnancy

Caution: uveitis

Side effects: ocular: red conjunctiva or lids, increased lash growth, increased iris pigmentation, increased peri-orbital pigmentation

Brimonidine (e.g., Alphagan P; topical, two to three times per day)

Indication: elevated IOP, premedication for laser eye surgery

Mechanism: α-receptor agonist, primarily α_2 (aqueous suppression and increased uveoscleral outflow)

Contraindication: concurrent use of monoamine oxidase inhibitors, children younger than 2 years (one drop may induce sedation for 24 hours)

Side effects: ocular: allergy, conjunctival injection; systemic: sedation, dizziness, dry mouth, decreased blood pressure

Brinzolamide (e.g., Azopt; topical, two to three times per day)

Indication: elevated IOP

Mechanism: carbonic anhydrase inhibitor (decreased aqueous production)

Contraindication: status-post corneal transplant surgery, kidney stones

Caution: compromised corneal endothelium

Side effects: ocular stinging and allergy, taste perversion (metallic taste)

Carbachol (e.g., Isopto Carbachol 0.75–3.0%; topical, three times per day) See **Pilocarpine** for indication, contraindication, side effects

Mechanism: both a direct acting cholinergic agonist and an indirect acting cholinergic by inhibiting acetylcholinesterase (increased outflow facility)

Ciprofloxacin (e.g., Ciloxin)

Indication: bacterial conjunctivitis, surgical infection prophylaxis

Mechanism: third-generation fluoroquinolone

Side effect: corneal toxicity

Cyclosporin A (e.g., Restasis; topical, twice per day)

Indication: moderate to severe dry eye, dry eye with associated blepharitis, status-post corneal transplant surgery

Mechanism: anti-inflammatory and immunomodulator that inhibits proliferation of inflammatory cells and activated T lymphocytes (stabilizes T lymphocytes)

Contraindication: current ocular infection

Side effects: ocular burning and stinging in 17% of patients, safe systemically

Cyclopentolate (e.g., Cyclogyl 0.5–2%, topical)

Indication: pupillary dilation (mydriasis), inhibiting accommodation (cycloplegia); for refracting pediatric patients or managing strabismus, deepen the anterior chamber (postoperative, e.g., after glaucoma surgery)

Mechanism: cholinergic antagonist at pupillary sphincter (mydriasis) and ciliary body (cycloplegia)

Contraindication: angle closure, albinos, infants, Down syndrome

Caution: pediatric patients (toxicity)

Side effects: urinary retention, tachycardia, delirium

Note: recovery: 24 hours

Diclofenac Sodium (e.g., Voltaren 0.1%, topical)

Indication: suppress pain and inflammation after cataract and laser surgery, temporary relief of pain and photophobia after corneal refractive surgery

Mechanism: nonsteroidal anti-inflammatory, inhibits cyclooxygenase

Caution: soft contact lens wear (irritation)

Side effects: keratitis, sterile corneal infiltrate, elevated IOP, dry eye complaints, inhibit wound healing

Dipivefrin (e.g., Propine; topical, twice a day)
Indication: elevated IOP
Mechanism: nonselective adrenergic agonist, primarily β_1 (initially aqueous suppression, then increased outflow facility)
Contraindication: aphakia, cystoid macular edema
Side effects: ocular: allergy, lid retraction, mydriasis (dilated pupils); systemic: tachycardia (less than epinephrine)

Dorzolamide (e.g., Trusopt; topical, two to three times a day)
Indication: elevated IOP
Mechanism: carbonic anhydrase inhibitor (decreased aqueous production)
Contraindication: status-post corneal transplant surgery, kidney stones
Caution: compromised corneal endothelium
Side effects: ocular stinging and allergy, taste perversion (metallic taste)

Dorzolamide hydrochloride timolol maleate (e.g., Cosopt, topical, one drop twice per day)
Combination Drug
Indication: elevated IOP
Mechanism: carbonic anhydrase inhibitor (decreased aqueous production) and non-selective beta blocker (decreased aqueous production)
Contraindication: post corneal transplant, kidney stones, asthma or reactive airway disease, bradycardia (check pulse before administration), arrhythmias, congestive heart failure, hypotension
Caution: compromised corneal endothelium
Side effects: ocular stinging and allergy, taste perversion, shortness of breath, dizziness, depression, impotence

Doxycycline (50–100 mg PO once or twice a day)
Indication: blepharitis, meibomian gland dysfunction, acne rosacea
Mechanism: reduces free fatty acid byproducts of meibomian gland secretions
Contraindication: pregnancy, children younger than 8 years (tooth discoloration)
Side effects: gastrointestinal upset, pseudotumor cerebri, skin sensitivity to light, hepatotoxicity

Echothiophate iodide (e.g., Phospholine Iodide 0.03%–0.25%; topical, twice a day)
Indication: elevated IOP, pupillary constriction (miosis)
Mechanism: indirect acting cholinergic by inhibiting cholinesterase (increased outflow facility)

Contraindication: narrow angles, uveitis

Side effects: blurred vision (especially younger patients or patients with cataract), brow ache, exacerbate iritis, exacerbate or precipitate angle closure glaucoma, retinal detachment

Note: Never use if general anesthesia planned with succinylcholine; combination may be fatal

Epinastine (e.g., Elestat 0.05%, topical, twice a day)

Indication: itching, allergic conjunctivitis

Mechanism: H_1 and H_2 receptor antagonist and mast cell stabilizer with anti-inflammatory activity

Side effects: constitutional symptoms

Epinephrine (topical)

Indication: elevated IOP

Mechanism: nonselective adrenergic agonist, primarily β_1 (initially aqueous suppression, then increased outflow facility)

Contraindication: aphakia, cystoid macular edema

Side effects: ocular: allergy, lid retraction, mydriasis (dilated pupils); systemic: tachycardia

Fluorometholone (e.g., FML 0.1%; topical)

Indication: anterior segment inflammation, conjunctivitis, cyclitis, dry eyes with/without blepharitis, after cataract surgery or keratoplasty, allergic conjunctivitis

Mechanism: anti-inflammatory inhibiting macrophages, neutrophils, and lymphocytes

Contraindication: herpes simplex or fungal keratitis

Side effects: elevated IOP (glaucoma), cataract (especially posterior subcapsular), secondary ocular inflammation

Note: less potent than prednisolone acetate

Gatifloxacin (e.g., Zymar, topical)

Indication: bacterial conjunctivitis, surgical infection prophylaxis

Mechanism: fourth-generation fluoroquinolone, better coverage for pseudomonas and atypical bacterias than third-generation fluoroquinolones

Side effects: corneal toxicity

Glycerine (e.g., Osmoglyn, 1.5–2 g/kg PO)

Indication: elevated IOP unresponsive to other medications, preoperative IOP reduction (not for chronic use)

Mechanism: osmotic

Contraindication: congestive heart failure, pulmonary edema, hypotension, concomitant use of another osmotic

Side effects: nausea and vomiting, congestive heart failure, hypotension, headache, dizziness, subarachnoid or subdural hemorrhage, mental confusion

Caution: diabetics (isosorbide may be better choice in diabetics)

Homatropine (topical)

> *Indication:* pupillary dilation (mydriasis), inhibiting accommodation (cycloplegia); for refracting pediatric patients or managing strabismus, deepen the anterior chamber (postoperative, e.g., glaucoma surgery)
>
> *Mechanism:* cholinergic antagonist at pupillary sphincter (mydriasis) and ciliary body (cycloplegia)
>
> *Contraindication:* angle closure, albinos, infants, Down syndrome
>
> *Caution:* pediatric patients (toxicity)
>
> *Side effects:* urinary retention, tachycardia, delirium
>
> *Note:* recovery: 1 to 3 days

Isosorbide (e.g., Ismotic, 1.5–2 g/kg PO)

> *Indication:* elevated IOP unresponsive to other medications, preoperative IOP reduction (not for chronic use)
>
> *Mechanism:* osmotic
>
> *Contraindication:* congestive heart failure, pulmonary edema, hypotension, concomitant use of another osmotic
>
> *Side effects:* congestive heart failure, hypotension, headache, dizziness, subarachnoid or subdural hemorrhage, mental confusion, nausea and vomiting (but less than glycerine)

Ketorolac tromethamine (e.g., Acular LS 0.4%, topical)

> *Indication:* suppress pain and inflammation after cataract and laser surgery, temporary relief of pain and photophobia after corneal refractive surgery, relief of itching from seasonal allergic conjunctivitis
>
> *Mechanism:* nonsteroidal anti-inflammatory, inhibits cyclooxygenase
>
> *Caution:* do not administer while wearing soft contact lenses (irritation)
>
> *Side effects:* keratitis, sterile corneal infiltrates, dry eye complaints, inhibits wound healing

Ketotifen fumarate (e.g., Zaditor, topical, twice per day)

> *Indication:* itching, allergic conjunctivitis
>
> *Mechanism:* H-1 receptor antagonist and mast cell stabilizer
>
> *Side effects:* conjunctival injection and constitutional symptoms

Latanoprost (e.g., Xalatan; topical, once at night)

> *Indication:* elevated IOP
>
> *Mechanism:* increased uveoscleral outflow (prostaglandin analog-hypotensive lipid, prostaglandin)
>
> *Contraindication:* cystoid macular edema, history of herpetic corneal disease, pregnancy
>
> *Caution:* uveitis
>
> *Side effects:* ocular: red conjunctiva or lids, increased lash growth, increased iris pigmentation, peri-orbital pigmentation

Levobunolol (e.g., Betagan 0.25–0.5%; topical, once or twice per day)

Indication: elevated IOP

Mechanism: nonselective beta blocker (decreased aqueous production)

Contraindication: asthma or reactive airway disease, bradycardia (check pulse before administration), arrhythmias, congestive heart failure, hypotension, third-degree heart block

Side effects: shortness of breath, dizziness, depression, impotence

Loteprednol etabonate (e.g., Alrex 0.2%, Lotemax 0.5%; topical)

Indication: anterior segment inflammation, conjunctivitis, cyclitis, dry eyes with/without blepharitis, after cataract surgery or keratoplasty, allergic conjunctivitis

Mechanism: anti-inflammatory inhibiting macrophages, neutrophils, and lymphocytes

Contraindication: herpes simplex or fungal keratitis

Side effects: elevated IOP (glaucoma, but less incidence than prednisolone acetate), cataract (especially PSC), secondary ocular inflammation

Note: less potent than prednisolone acetate, but associated with less risk of elevated IOP

Mannitol (1.5–2 g/kg IV over 1–1.5 hours)

Indication: elevated IOP unresponsive to other medications, preoperative IOP reduction

Mechanism: nonelectrolyte osmotic

Contraindication: congestive heart failure, pulmonary edema, hypotension, concomitant use of another osmotic

Side effects: congestive heart failure, hypotension, headache, dizziness, subarachnoid or subdural hemorrhage, mental confusion

Methazolamide (e.g., Neptazane 25–100 mg PO, three times per day) See **Acetazolamide**

Less efficacious and fewer side effects than acetazolamide

Moxifloxacin (e.g., Vigamox, topical)

Indication: Bacterial conjunctivitis, surgical infection prophylaxis

Mechanism: fourth-generation fluoroquinolone, better coverage for *Pseudomonas* and atypical bacteria than third-generation fluoroquinolones

Side effects: corneal toxicity

Ofloxacin (e.g., Ocuflox, topical)

Indication: bacterial conjunctivitis, surgical infection prophylaxis

Mechanism: third-generation fluoroquinolone

Side effects: corneal toxicity

Olopatadine HCL (e.g., Patanol 0.1%, topical, twice per day)
  Indication: itching, allergic conjunctivitis
  Mechanism: H_1 receptor antagonist and mast cell stabilizer
  Side effects: conjunctival injection and constitutional symptoms

Phenylephrine (e.g., Neo-Synephrine 2.5%, topical)
  Indication: pupillary dilation (mydriasis) for ophthalmoscopy, refraction (without cycloplegia), uveitis (prevent posterior synechia)
  Mechanism: α-adrenergic agonist, constrict radial muscles of iris (mydriasis only)
  Contraindication: narrow-angle or angle-closure glaucoma, significant cardiac disease or hypertension, sympathetic denervation (diabetics with neuropathy and patients on monoamine oxidase inhibitors)
  Side effects: arrhythmia and hypertension (usually with 10% solution)

Pilocarpine (e.g., Isopto Carpine 0.25–6.0%, topical, four times per day)
  Indication: elevated IOP, pupillary constriction (miosis)
  Mechanism: direct acting cholinergic agonist (increased outflow facility)
  Contraindication: narrow angles, uveitis
  Side effects: blurred vision (especially younger patients or patients with cataract), brow ache, exacerbate iritis, exacerbate or precipitate angle closure glaucoma, retinal detachment

Prednisolone acetate (e.g., Pred Forte 1%, topical)
  Indication: anterior segment inflammation, conjunctivitis, cyclitis, dry eyes with/without blepharitis, after cataract or glaucoma surgery or keratoplasty, allergic conjunctivitis
  Mechanism: anti-inflammatory inhibiting macrophages, neutrophils, and lymphocytes
  Contraindication: herpes simplex or fungal keratitis
  Side effects: elevated IOP (glaucoma), cataract (especially posterior subcapsular), secondary ocular inflammation
  Note: most potent topical steroid available

Prednisone (10–100 mg PO)
  Indication: scleritis, retinitis, vitritis, hyphema, optic neuritis (usually start with intravenous methylprednisolone)
  Mechanism: anti-inflammatory inhibiting macrophages, neutrophils, and lymphocytes
  Contraindication: tuberculosis, active systemic infection, pregnancy, peptic ulcer disease, psychosis
  Side effects: elevated IOP, cataract, hyperglycemia, hypertension, hypokalemia, psychosis, pseudotumor cerebri, inhibited wound healing, aseptic necrosis of bone, suppression of growth in children

Proparacaine (topical)

Indication: corneal anesthesia of short duration (e.g., for performing tonometry, gonioscopy, removal of corneal foreign body, anterior chamber paracentesis, cataract surgery)

Mechanism: stabilize the neuronal membrane, rendering it less permeable to ions

Contraindication: prolonged use, self-medication

Side effects: corneal epithelial erosions and ulcers with repeated and prolonged use

Rimexolone (e.g., Vexol; topical)

Indication: anterior segment inflammation, conjunctivitis, cyclitis, dry eyes with/without blepharitis, after cataract surgery or keratoplasty, allergic conjunctivitis

Mechanism: anti-inflammatory inhibiting macrophages, neutrophils, and lymphocytes

Contraindication: herpes simplex or fungal keratitis

Side effects: elevated IOP (glaucoma), cataract (especially posterior subcapsular), secondary ocular inflammation

Note: less potent than prednisolone acetate, but associated with less risk of elevated IOP

Scopolamine (e.g., Isopto Hyoscine 0.25%, topical)

Indication: pupillary dilation (mydriasis), inhibiting accommodation (cycloplegia); for refracting pediatric patients or managing strabismus, deepen the anterior chamber (postoperative, e.g., glaucoma surgery)

Mechanism: cholinergic antagonist at pupillary sphincter (mydriasis) and ciliary body (cycloplegia)

Contraindication: angle closure, albinos, infants, Down syndrome

Caution: pediatric patients (toxicity)

Side effects: urinary retention, tachycardia, delirium

Note: recovery: 3 to 7 days

Sodium chloride, hypertonic (e.g., Muro 128; topical or ointment, four times per day)

Indication: corneal edema

Mechanism: hyperosmotic (5% NaCl)

Side effects: burning and irritation

Tetracycline (250–500 mg PO, three to four times per day)

Indication: blepharitis, meibomian gland dysfunction, acne rosacea

Mechanism: reduces free fatty acid byproducts of meibomian gland secretion

Contraindication: pregnancy, children younger than 8 years (tooth discoloration)

Side effects: gastrointestinal upset, pseudotumor cerebri, skin sensitivity to light, hepatotoxicity

Timolol (e.g., Timoptic XE 0.25–0.5%; topical, once every morning)
  Indication: elevated IOP
  Mechanism: nonselective beta blocker (decreased aqueous production)
  Contraindication: asthma or reactive airway disease, bradycardia (check pulse before administration), arrhythmias, congestive heart failure, hypotension, third-degree heart block
  Side effects: shortness of breath, dizziness, depression, impotence

Travoprost (e.g., Travatan; topical, once every night)
  Indication: elevated IOP
  Mechanism: increased uveoscleral outflow (prostaglandin analog-hypotensive lipid, prostaglandin)
  Contraindication: cystoid macular edema, history of herpetic corneal disease, pregnancy
  Caution: uveitis
  Side effects: ocular: red conjunctiva or lids, increased lash growth, increased iris pigmentation, peri-orbital pigmentation

Tropicamide (e.g., Mydriacyl 0.5–1.0%, topical)
  Indication: pupillary dilation (mydriasis) for ophthalmoscopy, inhibiting accommodation (cycloplegia); for refracting pediatric patients or managing strabismus, uveitis (prevent posterior synechia)
  Mechanism: cholinergic antagonist at pupillary sphincter (mydriasis) and ciliary body (cycloplegia)
  Contraindication: angle closure, albinos, infants, Down syndrome
  Caution: pediatric patients (toxicity)
  Side effects: urinary retention, tachycardia, delirium
  Note: recovery: 4 to 6 hours

Unoprostone isopropyl (e.g., Rescula; topical, twice per day)
  Indication: elevated IOP
  Mechanism: increased outflow facility
  Contraindication: cystoid macular edema, history of herpetic corneal disease, pregnancy
  Caution: uveitis
  Side effects: ocular: red conjunctiva or lids, increased lash growth, increased iris pigmentation, periorbital pigmentation
  Note: Unoprostone isopropyl is less efficacious but associated with fewer side effects than other prostaglandin analogues-hypotensive lipids (i.e., Latanoprost, Bimatoprost, Travoprost)

D

Glossary

Abduction: movement of the eye temporally.

Accommodation: the increase in refractive power of the natural crystalline lens while doing near work.

Adduction: movement of the eye nasally.

Amaurosis fugax: blurred vision developing monocularly and lasting for minutes to hours. Hollenhorst plaques may be detected in retinal arteriol bifurcations.

Amblyopia: unilateral (or rarely bilateral) decrease in best-corrected central vision without visible evidence of an organic lesion corresponding to the level of visual loss.

Angle recession: cleavage in the ciliary body that splits between the longitudinal and circular muscle fibers; often a result of blunt trauma. May often result in secondary glaucoma.

Anisocoria: a difference in size between the two pupils. Usually greater than 2 mm.

Anisometropia: condition where the two eyes have a significant difference in refractive error (usually more than three diopters).

Anterior chamber: the space in the eye anterior to the pupil and iris and posterior to the cornea.

Astigmatism: the refractive power of the eye (cornea or lens) is not the same in all meridians (e.g., more myopia horizontally than vertically).

Bulbar conjunctiva: clear superficial covering of the globe extending from the limbus to the fornix.

Buphthalmos: enlargement of the globe secondary to elevated intraocular pressure in congenital glaucoma.

Cells (in anterior chamber): white blood cells (from inflammation), red blood cells (from trauma, hyphema), or pigmented cells (from retinal detachment or pigment dispersion) in the anterior chamber.

Chemosis: edema of the conjunctiva.

Coloboma: congenital absence of any eye structure in a particular location.

Conjunctivitis: inflammation of the conjunctiva.

Cotton-wool spot: infarction of the retinal ganglion cell layer appearing as a fluffy white lesion. Usually seen in hypertensive and diabetic retinopathy (also seen in other vascular occlusive disease).

Crowding phenomenon: letters are read better when presented individually as opposed to the whole line; most often seen in patients with amblyopia.

Cycloplegic: an agent that causes paralysis of the ciliary muscle with resultant paralysis of accommodation.

Descemet's membrane: basement membrane of the endothelial cells lining the posterior cornea.

Dilated fundus examination: examination of the retina, disc, and vitreous structures with an ophthalmoscope through a dilated pupil.

Diplopia: double vision.

Disc: optic nerve head.

Diurnal curve: multiple measurements of a patient's intraocular pressure (IOP) at different times throughout the day.

Ectopia lentis: dislocated lens.

Ectropion iridis: eversion of the iris at the pupil border resulting in visualization of the normally unseen pigmented posterior portion. Seen in diabetics with neovascularization of the iris.

Enophthalmos: state where globe is sunk into orbit (e.g. orbital fracture).

Enucleation: removal of the eye.

Episcleritis: inflammation of the external surface of the sclera underlying the bulbar conjunctiva.

Esophoria: latent deviation of the eye turning inward while not focusing; but eyes are aligned during binocular vision.

Esotropia: ocular misalignment where the nonfixating eye turns inward even when fixating with binocular vision.

Evisceration: surgical removal of the intraocular contents, while preserving the sclera and the extraocular muscle attachments.

Exenteration: excision of the eye and surrounding orbital contents.

Exophoria: latent deviation of the eye turning outward while not focusing; but eyes are aligned during binocular vision.

Exophthalmos: measurable protrusion of the globe from the orbit.

Exotropia: ocular misalignment where the nonfixating eye turns outward even when fixating with binocular vision.

Flare: elevated protein in the aqueous of the anterior chamber resulting in visualization of the slit lamp beam.

Flashes: transient visualization of light scintillations usually resulting from traction on the retina (vitreous detachment) or from a retinal detachment.

Floaters: visualized "dots" or "spots" that appear to shift location as the position of gaze is altered.

Fluorescein angiography: diagnostic test that utilizes intravenous fluorescein to demonstrate retinal pigment and retinal and choroidal vascular abnormalities; primarily performed to evaluate the posterior pole and macula.

Fovea: the center of the macula responsible for fine resolution and color vision.

Ghost vessels: blood vessels in the corneal stroma that do not contain blood.

Gonioscopy: study of the anterior chamber angle with a mirrored handheld lens applied to the cornea.

Guttata: central excrescences found on Descemet's membrane with increasing age and in conditions such as Fuch's dystrophy.

Haab's striae: breaks in Descemet's membrane as a result of elevated intraocular pressure in congenital glaucoma. Usually horizontal or concentric to the limbus.

Hard exudate: lipid deep in the retina demonstrating a yellow glistening appearance. Often a result of diabetic retinopathy.

Heterochromia: difference in coloration of the two irides of a patient.

Hyperopia (farsightedness): condition in which the eye cannot bring objects at distance and near into clear focus because the eye is too short or the refractive power is too weak.

Hyphema: blood in the anterior chamber as a clot or layered inferiorly. The term microhyphema describes suspension of blood cells in the anterior chamber.

Hypopyon: layering of white blood cells in the anterior chamber inferiorly.

Hypotony: intraocular pressure that is abnormally low (usually less than 6 mm Hg).

Indirect ophthalmoscopy: study of the fundus with a lens (usually a 20 or 28 diopter) held between the patient's eye and and the examiner in conjunction with a head-mounted light source.

Intraretinal microvascular abnormalities: retinal capillaries that are dilated (and often telangiectatic) acting as shunts between arterioles and venules.

Iritis (iridocyclitis, cyclitis, anterior uveitis): inflammation of the iris or ciliary body (or both) often manifested as an anterior chamber reaction.

Keratic precipitates: cellular debris (often inflammatory cells) that form on the corneal endothelium.

Krukenberg's spindle: a vertical band of pigment on the corneal endothelium. Usually, secondary to pigment dispersion.

Leukocoria: a white pupil.

Macula: posterior part of the retina about one disc diameter in size and centered at the fovea.

Meibomianitis: inflammation of the oil-bearing meibomian glands. The orifices just behind the lashes of the eyelids become inflamed and inspissated.

Microphthalmia: congenitally small and disorganized eye.

Miosis: constriction of the pupil.

Mydriasis: dilation of the pupil.

Myopia (nearsightedness): condition in which the eye cannot bring objects at distance into clear focus because the eye is too long or the refractive power too great.

Nanophthalmos: congenitally small eye that is otherwise normal.

Neovascularization: appearance of abnormal new blood vessels. Usually on the retina, optic nerve, or iris.

Nystagmus: rhythmic movement (tremors or oscillations) of the eyes that occur independently of normal eye movements.

Ophthalmoplegia: paralysis of the extraocular muscles.

Optic neuritis: inflammation of the optic nerve.

Ora serrata: most peripheral (and anterior) part of retina.

Oscillopsia: the perception that one's surroundings are moving back and forth.

Palpebral conjunctiva: clear superficial covering of the underside of the eyelids extending from the eyelid margins to the fornices.

Papilledema: bilateral swelling of the optic discs secondary to increased intracranial pressure.

Papillitis: inflammation of the optic nerve.

Peripapillary: area surrounding the optic disc.

Peripheral anterior synechia: adhesion between the peripheral iris and cornea obstructing the anterior chamber angle.

Peripheral iridectomy: removal of a section of the peripheral iris.

Phoria: latent tendency of the eyes to become misaligned (while not focusing); but under conditions of normal binocular vision, the eyes remain aligned.

Photophobia: ocular discomfort when exposed to light.

Photopsia: perception of instantaneous flashes of light.

Phthisis bulbi: condition in which the size of the eye is markedly reduced, the contents of the eye are completely disorganized, and the sclera is thickened.

Pinhole: aperture (ideally 1.2 mm) placed in front of the uncorrected eye (without glasses) during reading of the chart to determine if a refractive error (in the range −5 diopters to +5 diopters) is present.

Polycoria: presence of many openings in the iris stroma.

Posterior synechia: adhesion between the iris (usually pupillary border) and the anterior lens.

Proptosis: protrusion of the globe from the orbit.

Pseudohypopyon: layering of noninflammatory cells in the inferior anterior chamber, usually associated with neoplasia.

Ptosis: upper eyelid droop.

Punctum: opening of the tear-draining system along the eyelid margin.

Pupillary block: prevention of aqueous humor from flowing from the posterior chamber into the anterior chamber between the lens and iris.

Radial keratotomy: surgical procedure whereby radial incisions are made through 90% to 95% of the corneal stroma to flatten the corneal topography to reduce or eliminate myopia (nearsightedness).

Relative afferent pupillary defect: defect in the afferent parasympathetic pathway resulting in diminished constriction of the pupil with direct light. The consensual response remains intact.

Retinitis: inflammation of the retina.

Retinoscopy: a technique whereby the refractive error of the eye is estimated by observing the reflex from a streak of light shined on the retina.

Rhegmatogenous retinal detachment: retinal detachment secondary to a retinal tear (hole).

Sampoelesi's line: pigment deposition, scalloped in nature, anterior to Schwalbe's line. Seen by gonioscopy in pigment dispersion syndrome and pseudoexfoliation.

Scleral depression: technique in which the peripheral retina is observed by indirect ophthalmoscopy while peripheral retina is indented with an instrument held just posterior to the limbus.

Scleritis: inflammation of the sclera.

Scotoma: an area in the visual field where there is lost sensitivity.

Staphyloma: an outpouching (ectasia) of the sclera involving the uvea.

Strabismus: ocular misalignment.

Tarsorrhaphy: surgical technique in which the eyelid margins are surgically joined together.

Trabeculectomy: surgical technique to lower intraocular pressure by improving aqueous outflow in glaucoma patients.

Trichiasis: lash rubbing against the cornea.

Tropia: ocular misalignment even under conditions of normal binocular vision.

Vitritis: inflammation of the vitreous.

Aiello LM. Perspectives on diabetic retinopathy. Am J Ophthalmol 2003;136(1):122–135.

Beaver HA, Lee AG. The management of the red eye for the generalist. Compr Ther 2001;27(3):218–227.

Capao Filipe JA, Rocha-Sousa A, Falcao-Reis F, Castro-Correia J. Modern sports eye injuries. Br J Ophthalmol 2003;87(11):1336–1339.

Christoffersen NL, Larsen M. Pathophysiology and hemodynamics of branch retinal vein occlusion. Ophthalmology 1999;106(11):2054–2062.

Cunningham ET Jr, Belfort R Jr. HIV/AIDS and the Eye: A Global Perspective. San Francisco: Foundation of the American Academy of Ophthalmology, 2002.

Goldberg I. Relationship between intraocular pressure and preservation of visual field in glaucoma. Surv Ophthalmol 2003;48(2;suppl 1):S3–S7.

Klein R, Klein BE, Moss SE, Meuer SM. Retinal emboli and cardiovascular disease: the Beaver Dam Eye Study. Arch Ophthalmol 2003;121(10):1446–1451.

May DR, Kuhn FP, Morris RE, et al. The epidemiology of serious eye injuries from the United States Eye Injury Registry. Graefes Arch Clin Exp Ophthalmol 2000;238(2):153–157.

Monnet D, Breban M, Hudry C, et al. Ophthalmic findings and frequency of extraocular manifestations in patients with HLA-B27 uveitis. Ophthalmol 2004;111(4):802–809.

Nussenblatt RB, Whitcup SM, Palestine AG. Uveitis: Fundamentals and Clinical Practice. 2nd ed. St Louis: Mosby-Year Book, 1996.

Pieh C, Safran AB. Blockage of retrograde axonal flow after retinal artery occlusion: ophthalmoscopic findings. Arch Ophthalmol 2003;121(10):1508–1509.

Racette L, Wilson MR, Zangwill LM, et al. Primary open-angle glaucoma in blacks: a review. Surv Ophthalmol 2003;48(3):295–313.

Simon JW, Kaw P. Commonly missed diagnoses in the childhood eye examination. Am Fam Physician 2001;64(4):623–628.

Vafidis G. When is red eye not just conjunctivitis? Practitioner 2002;246(1636):469–471, 474–475, 478–481.

Vrabec TR. Posterior segment manifestations of HIV/AIDS. Surv Ophthalmol 2004;49(2):131–157.

Wilhelm H. Neuro-ophthalmology of pupillary function: practical guidelines. J Neurol 1998;245(9):573–583.

Index

Note: Page numbers with an f indicate figures; those with a t indicate tables; pl. indicates plate number.